Cultural Politics of Hygiene in India, 1890–1940

Cultural Politics of Hygiene in India, 1890–1940

Contagions of Feeling

Srirupa Prasad
University of Missouri–Columbia, USA

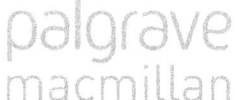

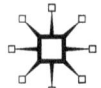

© Srirupa Prasad 2015

All rights reserved. No reproduction, copy or transmission of this publication may be made without written permission.

No portion of this publication may be reproduced, copied or transmitted save with written permission or in accordance with the provisions of the Copyright, Designs and Patents Act 1988, or under the terms of any licence permitting limited copying issued by the Copyright Licensing Agency, Saffron House, 6–10 Kirby Street, London EC1N 8TS.

Any person who does any unauthorized act in relation to this publication may be liable to criminal prosecution and civil claims for damages.

The author has asserted her right to be identified as the author of this work in accordance with the Copyright, Designs and Patents Act 1988.

First published 2015 by
PALGRAVE MACMILLAN

Palgrave Macmillan in the UK is an imprint of Macmillan Publishers Limited, registered in England, company number 785998, of Houndmills, Basingstoke, Hampshire RG21 6XS.

Palgrave Macmillan in the US is a division of St Martin's Press LLC, 175 Fifth Avenue, New York, NY 10010.

Palgrave Macmillan is the global academic imprint of the above companies and has companies and representatives throughout the world.

Palgrave® and Macmillan® are registered trademarks in the United States, the United Kingdom, Europe and other countries.

ISBN 978–1–137–52071–5

This book is printed on paper suitable for recycling and made from fully managed and sustained forest sources. Logging, pulping and manufacturing processes are expected to conform to the environmental regulations of the country of origin.

A catalogue record for this book is available from the British Library.

Library of Congress Cataloging-in-Publication Data
Prasad, Srirupa, 1971–
   Cultural politics of hygiene in India, 1890–1940 : contagions of feeling / Srirupa Prasad (University of Missouri–Columbia, USA).
      pages   cm. — (Cambridge imperial and post-colonial studies series)
      Summary: "Can there be an affective history of hygiene? Is it possible to read into the narrative of modern hygiene active and animated tropes of emotion, affect, and feeling? New microbes, novel pandemics, and their global movements that have forcefully reinstated the efficacy of hygiene have also reinvigorated global academic interest in the genealogies of hygienic practices. Cultural Politics of Hygiene in Bengal/India, 1890–1940 analyzes one such genealogy of hygiene in the context of late colonial Bengal. It argues that the meaning and role of hygiene in India were catalyzed on the crossroads of colonial governance, anticolonial struggles, cultural nationalism, and early 20th century social feminism. Affect, feeling, and sentiment were, however, no less important in the production of knowledge and practices of hygiene. Hygiene as a modern discourse, as shown in this book, not only produced emotions, sentiments, and feelings but was also constituted through them" — Provided by publisher.
   Includes bibliographical references.
   ISBN 978–1–137–52071–5 (hardback)
   1. Hygiene—Social aspects—India—Bengal—History. 2. Hygiene—Political aspects—India—Bengal—History. 3. Human body—Social aspects—India—Bengal—History. 4. Communicable diseases—Social aspects—India—Bengal—History. 5. Affect (psychology)—Social aspects—India—Bengal—History. 6. Public health—India—Bengal—History. 7. Bengal (India)—Social conditions—19th century. 8. Bengal (India)—Social conditions—20th century. 9. Bengal (India)—Colonial influence. 10. Bengal (India)—Politics and government. I. Title.
RA530.B4P73 2015
613.0954′14—dc23
                                          2015018341

Contents

List of Figures	vii
Acknowledgments	viii

1 Introduction: Contagion and Cultural Politics of Hygiene — 1
   Hygiene, colonialism, and affective histories — 5
   Objects, affect, and hygiene — 11
   Methods and sources — 17
   Outline of chapters — 20

2 Alimentary Anxieties: Affect in Food and Hunger — 23
   Histories of food and the body — 26
   Food adulteration, embodiment, and the politics of anxiety — 27
   Famine's bodies — 33

3 Body, Hygiene, and the Affective Politics of Gandhi's *Swaraj* — 43
   Body, affect, and Gandhi — 46
   Gandhi's fasts — 50
   Race and Gandhi's politics of hygiene — 52
   Medicine as contagion — 56

4 Imagining the Social Body: Competing Moralities of Care and Contagion — 60
   Locating women's writings on care in early twentieth-century India — 62
   Memorable objects: Childhood, memory, and care in Shukhalata Rao's writings — 66
   Memorable spaces: Suffering and education of care in Priyabala Gupta's memoir — 75
   Traveling memories: Wandering and care in Purnashashi Debi's autobiography — 81

5 Affective Remedies: Advertisements and Cultural Politics of Hygiene 89
Enchantments of empire and nation 91
Advertising, consumer culture, and empire 94
Advertisements and a pluralist medical marketplace 96
Advertising beauty, womanhood, and domesticity 102
Contagion of advertisements 109

Conclusion 113

Notes 117

References 130

Index 138

Figures

5.1 Page of a newspaper from 1898 showing the advertisements of medical products from a variety of medical knowledge systems *Amrita Bazar Patrika*, February 10, 1898   98

5.2 Advertisement of Jabakusum Hair Oil from *Grihasthamangal*, May 28, 1928   104

Acknowledgments

It has taken me a while to give this book its final shape. While the writing of the book happened over a relatively short time, its conceptualization has had a much longer history. And, needless to say, this process could be sustained because of generous emotional, intellectual, and institutional support. Writing acknowledgments is therefore tough, and there is a risk of missing out someone who has contributed to the book in one way or another. Any omission is completely unintended.

First, I would like to express my gratitude toward two people without whom this book simply would not have seen the light of day – my mentor Antoinette Burton and my husband Amit Prasad. I cannot thank them enough for their incredible support – in more ways than one – during the writing of this book. Antoinette read each of the chapters, and at times several versions of them, and provided critical feedback. I cherish our regular Skype conversations during the writing of this book. As always, Amit was an astute reader and critic of this book, reading every bit, offering valuable comments, and rewriting passages.

I am grateful to my friends Rebecca Scott, Sarasij Majumdar, and Satadru Sen who read parts of the manuscript and gave me feedback.

My writing sessions with Debarati Sen, Donna Strickland, and Tara Pauliny were of invaluable help during those long summer afternoons when, at times, it seemed that the book might never be completed. Donna provided very useful insights into the craft of writing.

The main archival research for this book was made possible by funding from the Wenner-Gren Foundation for Anthropological Research. A Summer Research Fellowship and a Research Board Grant from the University of Missouri funded additional archival research.

I would like to warmly thank Joan Hermsen for all her advice and help. I would like to express my gratitude to Ibitola Pearce and Jay Gubrium, my departmental mentors. Linda Reeder and Devoney Looser gave valuable suggestions. Thank you Jenna Pirok and Katie Knop for your research assistance. I truly value the caring friendship and encouragement of Mary Jo Neitz. Thank you for being there. I have also cherished knowing and interacting with my other colleagues in the departments of Women's & Gender Studies and Sociology at the University of Missouri.

I owe a great deal to the wonderful editors at Palgrave Macmillan. Thank you Jade Moulds and Jenny McCall for your incredible assistance in giving shape to this book and your endless patience. I owe a special note of thanks to Ashok Ravi and the copyeditor/s. I cannot thank them enough for their keen scrutiny of the manuscript and immensely helpful suggestions and corrections.

Parts of this book were presented at several workshops and conferences and have benefited tremendously from the feedback. I would like to especially thank Ishita Pande, Tirthankar Roy, Akio Tanabe, Takashi Oishi, Madhulika Banerjee, Kirin Narayan, Simona Sawhney, and Deepak Kumar. I am grateful to my colleagues at the University of Wisconsin–Madison. In particular, I would like to thank Warwick Anderson, Judy Houck, Judith Leavitt, and Ronald Numbers for their useful suggestions and support. Sanjay Bhattacharya has been immensely supportive and offered valuable feedback in the early stages of my research.

This book arose from my dissertation research, which would not have been possible without the generous support of Winifred Poster, Jan Nederveen Pieterse, Moon-Kie Jung, Charis Thompson, Zsuzsa Gille, Michael Goldman, Zine Magubane, Maneesha Desai, Maneesha Lal, Paula Treichler, and Antoinette Burton. It would not have been possible also without the friendship and help of grad school friends – Indranil Dutta, Tulsi Dharmarajan, Emin Adas, Serife Genis, Himika Bhattacharya, and Danielle Kinsey.

The journey of this book also owes a great deal to my friends, especially Sarbari Dasgupta, Sam Bullington, and Niharika Banerjea.

I would like to especially thank Ashim Mukhopadhyay of the National Library, Kolkata (formerly Calcutta), for offering precious help during my work there. The librarians of the Asian and African Studies Collection at the British Library offered much help in accessing books and journals. Doing archival research for this book at the Centre for Studies in Social Sciences, Calcutta, has been undoubtedly the most memorable part of my research. I wish to especially thank Abhijit Bhattacharya, Indira Biswas, Prabir Roy, and Kamalika Mukherjee who have no idea how much they have contributed to this book. During the early years of this research project, Indira Chowdhury and Sudeshna Banerjee helped me immensely with archival sources, especially on domesticity and health.

Thank you Maroona Murmu. I learned much from you about the history of Bengali women's autobiographies and you will always remind me of our long hours of grind in the archives. It was a lot of fun.

I have also learned much from my discussions with Pradip Kumar Bose, Gautam Bhadra, and Tapati Guha Thakurta, particularly with regard to nineteenth- and twentieth-century archives of Bengal's cultural history.

I would like to thank Janaki Nair and Tanika Sarkar for their valuable suggestions.

I wish to thank my family, especially my brother, who was always eager to know about the progress of the book whenever we talked on the phone.

Finally, I would like to thank Zara, my lifeline. Watching you fetch the ball tirelessly has taught me a great deal about mindfulness and persistence. You continue to create magic every day.

1
Introduction: Contagion and Cultural Politics of Hygiene

Hygiene is back in the headlines. In slightly more than a decade, the SARS outbreak, the swine flu, and more recently the avian flu have created panic across the globe, forcing people to take notice of contagions that could turn deadly and infect scores of people in a relatively short time. The world suddenly became a shared landscape of closely linked contact zones that are teeming with hundreds of potent microbes, which do not care about national or cultural boundaries.

This shift, understandably, has resulted in a spate of writings on the precariousness of the global population. Experts and non-experts alike have emphasized our alarming susceptibility to new forms of microbial infections. Science writers and journalists, notably Richard Preston, Laurie Garrett, Barry and David Zimmerman, and David Quammen, have published sensational and dramatic titles on the topic. And some of these, for example, *The Hot Zone: A Terrifying True Story*; *The Demon in the Freezer*; *The Coming Plague: Newly Emerging Diseases in a World Out of Balance*; and *Betrayal of Trust: The Collapse of Global Public Health* have became best sellers and are being taught in courses on public and global health and international security.[1] These writings, highlighting the dangers of new and tougher microbes, discuss covert laboratory projects in the United States, and rogue nations storing deadly microbes that could be used against that and other nations, and they argue for freezing viruses that could come handy in times of war.

Even seminal medical journals such as *The Lancet* and *The New England Journal of Medicine* have adopted a distinct tone of urgency in discussing illnesses like the common flu and the role of viruses that are mutating into newer forms and becoming more formidable each day. The US-based Centers for Disease Control (CDC) and Prevention now publishes a journal called *Emerging Infectious Diseases*. This growing body of articles, books, media reports, and policy guidelines on global preparedness in the face of new infectious diseases reflects the emergence of an important debate and a major governmental endeavor in health and medicine that has global reach.

India has zealously joined this new endeavor. The call for better hygiene has brought together a number of forces and institutions in the management of sanitation in India. The Indian government, along with non-governmental Indian organizations, international and national academic institutions, multinational companies, and global philanthropic enterprises such as the Bill and Melinda Gates Foundation, have embarked upon what are termed public–private initiatives to promote public health. Since 2006, the Global Hygiene Council, an organization funded by Reckitt Benckiser (famous for its antiseptic product, Dettol), has, for example, undertaken a campaign to bring together private and public initiatives to promote awareness of hygiene and personal sanitation, especially among the economically weaker sections of the population. This initiative has marked a new phase in the current public health agenda in India. It has mobilized public and private entities and resources to ameliorate the poor state of institutional capacity and sought to direct its focus on improvements in the teaching, research, and policy of public health. One of its campaigns, the Dettol *Surakshit Parivar* (Dettol Protected Family), was designed to educate new mothers, students, and hospital workers about one of the most important aspects of personal and collective hygiene – washing hands to prevent infection by germs.

Another influential entity in this enterprise, The Public Health Foundation of India (PHFI), was launched in 2006 as 'a response to redress the limited institutional capacity in India for strengthening training, research and policy development in the area of Public Health'.[2]

> Structured as an independent foundation, PHFI adopts a broad, integrative approach to public health, tailoring its endeavours to Indian conditions and bearing relevance to countries facing similar challenges and concerns. The PHFI focuses on broad

dimensions of public health that encompass promotive, preventive and therapeutic services, many of which are frequently lost sight of in policy planning as well as in popular understanding.³

Hygiene has undoubtedly attracted a lot of attention in India, as in the rest of the world, as being the cornerstone for a robust program in public health for the twenty-first century. It has become a sociologically significant phenomenon in which global concerns are being managed by simultaneously roping in a number of actors and institutions, ranging from the nation-state to the family. New microbes, novel pandemics, and their global movements that have forcefully reinstated the efficacy of hygiene have also reinvigorated global academic interest in the genealogies of hygienic practices.

This book analyzes one such genealogy of hygiene in the context of late colonial Bengal. It argues that the meaning and role of hygiene in India were catalyzed on the crossroads of colonial governance, anti-colonial struggles, cultural nationalism, and early twentieth-century feminism. As a consequence of a variety of historical processes – political, economic, social, and cultural – engagement with hygiene not only shifted public health discourse in the early twentieth century, it also produced hygiene as a set of practices that guided gendered domestic agendas in Bengal. These domestic agendas included guidelines for preparation of food, care of sick patients, childcare, and patterns of domestic consumption of drugs and beauty products.

Spencer Harcourt Butler, a member of the Department of Education in the Governor General's Council, highlighted these issues while presiding over the second All India Sanitary Conference, which opened its session at the Council Chamber, Fort St. George, Madras, in November 1912. The need for a broader partnership and persistent efforts at better hygiene was also not lost on Butler:

> Ideas and interests have been quickened on all sides and there are signs of a sanitary awakening in India, of the dawning of an age of greater attention to public health... You, I know, will not fail, gentlemen, when the call for the expert resounds throughout this ancient land. We specially welcome the presence of non-official representatives of the different provinces as an augury of that co-operation between experts and laymen, without which as I pointed out last year, it will be difficult if not impossible, to

achieve any widespread sanitary progress in this country... You, I know, will not fail, gentlemen, when the call for the expert resounds throughout this ancient land; and, meanwhile, you will push forward the work to which you have laid your hands with dauntless patience and indefatigable zeal.

(1912:1)

In fact, by the early years of the twentieth century, colonial governance showed a degree of urgency with regard to sanitation that was unprecedented. The first All India Annual Sanitary Conference started in 1911, and by 1912, despite some differences of opinion, one thing was unanimously agreed upon – sanitary reform was the most important agenda facing the colonial Indian government at that time. The language that was used to express this concern left little doubt about the importance that the colonial rulers of India attached to the cause of sanitation. The phrase 'sanitary awakening' not only referred to a state of governance within which the cause of sanitation was given a fresh lease of colonial urgency, but also to a new form of 'consciousness', a new moral-political realization, which could bring about a very different order of social transformation and become another element of the civilizing mission. Not surprisingly, sanitation, for colonial officials, was equal in standing to, if not more important than, medical research as a means for progress in medicine and health.[4]

The Cultural Politics of Hygiene is a study of the emergence of hygiene as a socially and medically useful knowledge and practice in India and its intertwined relationship with cultural and social transformation in colonial Bengal. It shows how hygiene emerged from within the colonial governance and political engagements of the Bengali middle class, and through a focus on the formation of modern and cultured subjectivities.

The book analyzes how and why hygiene became authoritative and succeeded in becoming a part of the broader social and cultural vocabulary within colonialist, anti-colonial, and modernist discourses. In particular, it investigates how the emergence of hygiene as a powerful ideology, knowledge, and practice redefined and reconfigured two of the most influential realms of social life in early twentieth-century Bengal – the household and the nation. It argues that hygiene emerged and materialized within the domestic and the national realm around two intertwined and mutually reinforcing axes: the emergence and arrangement of objects, commodities, and things; and affect.

The emergence of hygiene took place through the accelerated production, availability, and visibility of a wide range of commodities and things. Medicines, cosmetics, household goods, and food items opened up a whole new way of imagining and practicing hygiene. The history of hygiene will remain incomplete if this dense realm of commodities and things is not taken into account in the very active sense of producing the meaning and values of modern hygiene. New ideas and practices about cleanliness, nursing, and nutrition emerged, for example, in specific relation to a flourishing market of commodities.

Affect, feeling, and sentiment were, however, no less important in the production of the knowledge and practices of hygiene. Hygiene as a modern discourse, as I show in this book, not only produced emotions, it was also constituted through them. In fact, it would not be an exaggeration to say that hygiene worked effectively by attributing emotions to a range of practices, involving both the individual (citizen, householder, neighbor) and the collective (social, cultural, and national) body. Disgust, fear, anxiety, and pain, for example, were (and continue to be) important markers in defining health and wellbeing.

Hygiene, colonialism, and affective histories

Can there be an affective history of hygiene? In other words, is it possible to read into the narrative of modern hygiene active and animated tropes of emotion, affect, and feeling? In what ways can such a reading of archives on hygiene and public health offer us a more complex and layered understanding of the paradoxical and conflicted ways in which this 'tool of empire' functioned?

In this book, I argue that affect was indispensable and integral to chronicles of public health and hygiene in late colonial India. Affect, emotion, and feelings produced an impressive template for cleanliness, care, and order for the modern Indian nation, society, and household. Such a template, I further argue, is not merely a glaze on the more serious content of the public health and sanitary documents of the British Empire; it constitutes the very basis of this colossal archive and the ideas and practices it mandated. The archives of hygiene in colonial India direct us to the depths and 'hidden forces' of, to borrow a phrase from Ann Laura Stoler, and the 'epistemic anxieties and colonial common sense' that guided public health endeavors in colonial India. That is, these archives present 'a display of sentiments that evinced more powerful mystic and mental states'.[5]

A focus on affective tropes of hygiene opens up a 'moving' history of the Empire and its huge apparatus, which churned out countless ideas, documents, and aspirations.[6] By 'moving' I mean the trials, shifts, failures, frustrations, and fears that characterized the gestation, deliberation, administration, and documentation of hygiene, public health, and sanitation in late colonial India. I use the term 'moving' also to highlight the dynamic relationship of the prescriptions of health and hygiene with the sensibilities of their prescribers. Modern hygiene was thus as much a set of instructions for bodily health, moral sanctions, and cultural prescriptions for individuals and society, as it was an embodiment of the intellectual, emotional, and imaginative sensibilities of those who professed and wrote about them.

Contagions of Feeling excavates the moving history of modern hygiene by exploring the affective trajectories of public health as they were defined, designed, appropriated, and manipulated for the needs of the British Empire in late colonial India. Indians did not blindly follow the sensibilities and goals of the colonial rulers, however. They, in particular educated Indians, vigorously discoursed about health and hygiene and tied these concerns in with nationalism, self-rule, and modernity.

'Contagion' and 'feeling' are central elements in the moving history of hygiene in colonial India that I present in this book. I focus on contagion to signify the interconnected impact of a wide range of activities that encapsulated public health and sanitation in colonial India. The narratives of public health in colonial India were surely not all about infectious diseases, quarantine, and emergency sanitary administration. Public health was equally about non-emergency, yet essential activities, such as policing market places, maintaining vital statistics of populations, and quality control of food and water. These domains of hygiene and public health were entwined in their concern with transmission, and, consequently, infection and pestilence caused by contagions. The concept of contagion was thus significant in a number of ways.

Public health in colonial India can be traced back to the primary concern, as historians of medicine have convincingly shown, with the health and safety of British troops in India.[7] Over time and with the further consolidation of the British Empire, medicine diversified into a wide range of colonial activities that spanned research, teaching, and other organizational work, epitomized by the highly colonial-bureaucratic Indian Medical Service (IMS), for example.[8] Yet it would not be an exaggeration to argue that infection and contagion always loomed as a menace that could erupt anytime unless vigilantly kept under control. The colonial state had to keep in mind that infectious diseases such as cholera, plague, and smallpox were huge financial burdens and these, at extreme moments, could grind the entire administration to a halt as experiences during the worst epidemics had shown.

In addition, and no less important, was another worry that was voiced urgently at the international sanitary conferences – how international trade was badly impacted by epidemics and the resultant quarantines. Contagion thus remained the shadowy but real threat that was at the heart of colonial sanitary administration during the entire tenure of the British Empire in India. If one reflects on the more recent history of public health globally, one cannot fail to notice how rapid disease transmission, the affliction of large populations, and the impact of these on global economy and trade still remain the major concern for the global public health community.

Priscilla Wald, for example, provides a fascinating account of the dominant 'outbreak narrative' that ensues when an infectious disease breaks out in the post-HIV world. She shows that this particular narrative trope gained prominence in the post-HIV era through a predictable combination of 'particular characters, images, and story lines – of Patients Zero and superspreaders, hot zones and tenacious microbes'.[9] Tracing this 'outbreak narrative' to 'U.S. economic and political dominance in the institutionalization of ideas about global health worldwide', Wald argues that its 'circulation across genres and media makes it at once the reflection and the structuring principle of scientific and journalistic accounts, novelistic and cinematic depictions of communicable-disease outbreaks, and even the contemporary proliferation of historical studies of the central role of communicable disease in human history'.[10] I find Wald's idea of 'outbreak narratives' very useful, especially the way she deploys it to excavate the cultural terrain of twentieth-century America. She shows convincingly how science and myth are inseparable, the social and the biological are interlinked, and how fiction and other cultural productions are the sources of some of the most authoritative scientific narratives of our times.

I present contagion as an analytical centerpiece also by drawing upon the scholarship in history of medicine in the context of colonial India. Medicine, for colonial officials such as Butler, whose ideas of sanitary awakening I briefly discussed earlier, was a means for social change and therefore could not be realized if it was pursued only within the walls of medical laboratories. Medicine was to be ably served by scientists and doctors as much as by administrators such as Butler or Lukis (the Surgeon General at that time). The concern for these colonial officers was not simply the therapeutic and curative implications of medicine. Rather, for them, health and medicine symbolized advanced forms of collective social life. One must take note of the fact, however, that the sheer magnitude of this task made it impossible for experts or administrators alone to realize it. This exigency of management made it imperative to give a clarion call to Indians to come together with colonial rulers in this sanitary mission, which, although taken up by Indians, did not imply convergence of goals.

I focus on Butler's address to the All India Sanitary Conference also because of the other important connection that it sought to forge – between 'experts' and their work in the service of what Butler called the 'ancient land' of India. The phrase 'ancient land' embodies the tension that characterized liberal reformist agendas of the British Empire in the late nineteenth and early twentieth centuries. The opening speech of Butler was thus striking not only in its implications in terms of ideas for action, regeneration, and progress, but also in revealing the philosophical and ideological premises of much of British liberal political thought that undergirded imperial projects.

Uday Mehta and Thomas Metcalf have highlighted this tension with great clarity. They argue that liberalism was truly a radical philosophy, which sought to draw the limits of state intervention in the lives of individual citizens, and to that extent it carried with itself doctrines of universalism, suffrage, and self-representation.[11] Yet in its historical actualization in the colonies, liberalism not only kept groups of people and societies outside the purview of its universal claims, it in fact became a tool that concealed disenfranchisement and marginalization in the garb of ultimate greater good.

The transposition of 'ancient land' and 'expert' exemplified this contradiction: the ancient land, which signified the outmoded institutions and social practices in India, could thus be regenerated by proper knowledge and under the watchful eyes of (British/Western) experts. Only good governance, enshrined in the doctrines of modern knowledge and Western benevolence, could usher a social transformation that would bring the 'ancient land' out of the stupor of age-old hierarchical customs and into the age of self-rule. The claim for the universal possibility of social transformation was always questionable when it concerned colonized societies who were yet to be as 'civilized' as British society.

This philosophical and ideological climate undergirded the dominant colonial agenda in late colonial Bengal/India and was implemented through a mix of eighteenth-century European medical policing, the nineteenth-century model of large-scale public health initiatives, and the rudiments of twentieth-century consciousness around preventive medicine and hygiene. Overall, colonial health policies had two crucial imperatives – one military and the other missionary.[12] While military interest served as the blueprint for most colonial governments' undertakings in public health and sanitary projects in the presidency cities and other urban centers, the missionary ethic or 'clinical Christianity' gained favor in relation to preventive medicine and for personal hygiene and sanitation.[13]

Poonam Bala, highlighting the inordinate delay in the establishment of public health priorities in colonial India and their subservience to British commercial interests, has argued that while the army was last on the British health agenda, in the context of colonial India, it was just the reverse.[14] Bala contends that after the 1857 mutiny and subsequent takeover of the Empire by the Crown, army health became the prime concern of the colonial health policy, which was entrusted to the hands of the IMS. Radhika Ramasubban, similarly, argues that the health of the wider colonized population was compromised at the expense of the medical needs of the colonial military.[15]

Although some historians have contested a straightforward link between medical priorities in colonial India and the interests of the military, there is a consensus among scholars working on colonial

India that army health was the motivating force behind colonial health policies.[16] David Arnold, for example, shows how 'colonial enclavism' and excessive attention given to the military and its health requirements limited the scope of many public health initiatives before 1900. '[T]he continuing narrowness of official preoccupations', Arnold writes, 'was reflected in the annual reports of the sanitary commissioners in the 1870s which devoted 80 or 90 pages to the health of European soldiers, but less than a dozen each to the "native" army, prisoners, and the "general population"'.[17]

The Contagious Diseases Acts, which required forceful inspection of prostitutes serving the military, became another exemplification of the predominant concern for the army in colonial India. Anil Kumar shows how Lock hospitals served the 'twin purposes of facilitating mercenary sex and protecting the soldiers from the infections of venereal diseases'.[18] The health crisis of the army following the Crimean War further consolidated the military focus of the healthcare system. Interestingly, this crisis in the army's health prompted Florence Nightingale to comment on the absolute necessity for a public health re-awakening for a country that she described as the 'land of domestic filth' and a 'focus of epidemics'. The cleverness of Nightingale, as Mary Poovey argued, lay in the way she deployed the ideal of 'care' to support Britain's imperial designs in India.[19]

The plague of 1896–1897 eventually stirred Indians as well as the colonial government to take notice of the enormity of public health concerns in India.[20] 'The discovery of the dreaded bubonic plague in Bombay City in September 1896', Prashant Kidambi writes, 'precipitated a political and social crisis unknown in colonial India since 1857'.[21] There was a spurt in sanitary activities following the plague. Preventive measures to control epidemics were consequently looked at more favorably and an urgent need for health education in the wider population was emphasized. Contagion, infection, and disease transmission conveyed not only the predicaments of a besieged colonial state in relation to health of Indians, there was also intense international pressure given the commercial importance of the affected area.[22] The term 'pathogenic' thus acquired meaning and value through an interweaving of the medical and the social. The 'intermingling of social and scientific theories of contagion', as Priscilla Wald argues in a different context, also 'led to the articulation of a form of collective identity and a principle of belonging that is at the heart of the outbreak narrative'.[23]

The main objective of *Contagions of Feeling* is to show that the formation and vitality of any form of knowledge and practice are intrinsically tied to the affective worldings of particular communities. Moreover, given that social groups are defined by and rest on different codes of exclusion and inclusion such as gender, class, caste, or religion, ideas and practices of hygiene commonly exemplify these exclusions (and inclusions). At the heart of anxieties about microbial contagion lay apprehensions about social and moral belonging. Social, cultural, and ultimately moral contamination produced the same kinds of menace that pestilence did. These anxieties were germane to the production of discourses on disease, health, and body in colonial Bengal and India more broadly. Affect in this context was the catalyst that translated pestilence, filth, and disease into a socially and culturally authorized vocabulary of purity, pollution, and cleanliness.

Affective textures of contagion thus not only spread across a wide range of discourses and practices, they also continually grow as affects themselves become contagious. 'Thinking of affects as contagious', Sara Ahmed explains, helps 'us to challenge an "inside out" model of affect by showing how affects pass between bodies, affecting bodily surfaces or even how bodies surface'. However, as Ahmed elaborates, 'affective contagion tends to underestimate the extent to which affects are contingent... affect becomes an object only given the contingency of how we are affected, or only as an effect of how objects are given'.[24]

This book examines genealogies of contagion in colonial Bengal/India and thereby explores the dynamic and contested passages between contagion as microbe and contagion as affect. It analyzes epistemic, material, cultural, and affective dimensions of contagion to open up entanglements of empire and nation, power and difference, modernity and tradition.

Objects, affect, and hygiene

Despite the depth of intellectual engagement with hygiene, historians have not explored the ways in which specific objects and commodities embody (and are made distinct by) certain affects and the ways in which these objects become meaningful as cultural productions in the context of health and medicine. It is, therefore, imperative to explore the affective histories that objects and commodities engendered in the lives and imaginations of middle class consumers in late colonial Bengal.

In the late nineteenth and early twentieth centuries certain objects became particularly charged with emotions and feelings about the empire, national belonging, cultural identity, and economic self-sustenance. These objects became animated with particular affects and feelings as the medical marketplace became flooded with promises of cures and wellbeing. The affective charge of objects often crossed over to, and was further animated by, debates on the British Empire, Indian nationalism, and political self-rule in India. These objects and commodities were thus instrumental in making hygiene/cleanliness a vital ingredient in debates on cultural and political self-fashioning. In this book, I delve into the mutual production of objects, commodities, and affect as a robust site of, and mechanism for the production of hygiene as a discourse that warranted a set of cultural practices.

The objects and commodities I focus on relate to health and wellbeing. Cures for a range of common ailments, products used for cleanliness and disinfection, and specialty food for children and the sick collectively created a thriving medical-therapeutic-curative marketplace in the late nineteenth and the early twentieth centuries. This complex set of commodities and objects was instrumental in making hygiene, purity, and moral cleanliness vital elements of debates on cultural and political self-fashioning. More specifically, I explore four inter-related processes: (1) the commodification of medical and hygienic products in late colonial India, (2) the 'pluralism' that characterized the medical marketplace in India, (3) the gendered nature of the new commodity consciousness, and (4) the linkages between ideologies and practices of different institutions and socio-political structures that together defined medical consumerism in Bengal/India during this period.

In the late nineteenth and the early twentieth centuries Bengali (as well as other Indian language) and English newspapers and magazines became competitive advertising places where allopathic, homeopathic, Ayurvedic, electrotherapeutic, and *hakimi* nostrums vied for legitimacy. Advertisements in Victorian England also offered medical assistance through a combination of pills, electrical treatment, and surgery. However, their counterparts in Bengal/India offered not only a multiplicity of cures within the allopathic tradition, but also a plurality of other medical therapies as well: *Unani*, Ayurveda, and homeopathy successfully competed against allopathic medicines and practices. Homeopathy, although not a native medical tradition, became immensely popular in urban Bengal.[25] David Arnold and Sumit Sarkar have argued that homeopathic treatment found increasing favor among urban Bengalis because it was cheap and easy to use, and because it was not associated with British colonial authority.[26]

In short, the medical marketplace in colonial India/Bengal was a site of contested knowledges and practices in which a number of medical systems seriously challenged the monopoly of allopathic drugs and cures. This was also significant because the late nineteenth and early twentieth centuries presented a regeneration of the existing medical knowledges and practices of Bengal. This was also the period when the colonial state pursued an active and aggressive policy of professionalization and regulation in Bengal that was productively utilized by Indian businessmen.[27] Ayurveda, for example, was given fresh impetus by enthusiasts such as Gangaprasad Sen, Neelamber Sen, and Gangadhar Ray, who were inspired to undertake large scale production by establishing the pharmaceutical company N.N. Sen and Company Private Limited.

Similar efforts were made to commercialize Ayurvedic drugs. In 1901 several pharmaceutical companies, for example Dhaka Oushadhalaya, Sadhana Oushadhalaya, and Kalpataru Ayurvedic Works, were established and they soon became successful.[28] Another well-known pharmaceutical company, Bengal Chemicals and Pharmaceutical Works Limited, was established in 1901 through the pioneering efforts of Acharya Prafulla Chandra Ray. This particular company was the first drug company completely owned and managed by Indians. One particular factor that contributed to the growth of the Indian therapeutic market was the disruption caused by World War I. The War led to a drastic decline in imports and Indian companies used this opportunity to spur local production.

The thriving medical market gained foothold through aggressive advertising and in this it relied on the vibrant and growing print capitalism in colonial India. In fact, the domain of medical-hygienic-therapeutic advertisements constitutes one of the most productive sites to explore the negotiations of a host of material and epistemological issues that were crucial in charting out the contours of medical practice in late colonial India. While semantically dense and culturally meaningful in their own accord, in colonial India, these advertisements were also a part of a broader milieu that bridged political practices of the state, the household, and the civil-public sphere.

The Indian medical marketplace has often been characterized as representing, to use E.D. Ackernecht's phrase, a 'therapeutic chaos'.[29] It was, in fact, a vibrant and pluralistic market that consisted of a plethora of curative products and possibilities. The gradual shift of the British colonial state's policy in favor of an anti-contagionist and sanitarianist-environmentalist approach to public health, popular protests against the colonial government's quarantine policies, and a truly favorable response by Indians only in matters of surgery, had amply demonstrated that the monopoly of biomedicine was far from complete. Popular protests against the colonial government's health initiatives did not imply chaos. Rather, they often represented critiques of colonial rule, which were also utilized by Indians to further pluralistic medical ideologies and practices. It was thus no coincidence that hygiene as a mechanism to re-think and re-organize both the corporeal and the ideological body of the nation found a truly appropriate moment during this period: a moment that Joseph Alter has aptly called a time of 'somatic nationalism'.[30]

In *Contagions of Feeling*, as discussed earlier, I locate affect at the heart of circulations of commodities/objects/things and their social, political, and cultural worldings. The affective becomes particularly forceful when commodities, and more broadly commodity culture, end up inhabiting charged economic and political times and spaces. In this regard the book is located within a compelling body of scholarship in history, anthropology, and literary and cultural studies that has explored the social, economic, and cultural lives of commodities, objects, and things in the contexts of colonialism and empire. Historians and anthropologists have, for example, chronicled the rich history of commodities and, more broadly, Indian markets in the colonial and postcolonial period. Tea, cotton, indigo, and opium are some of the items studied by these scholars. One particular commodity that has been frequently explored for its economic, social, cultural, and political significance has been Khadi – the handspun and hand woven cloth that is derived from cotton.[31] Khadi or khaddar achieved an iconic status in the anti-colonial struggle when Mahatma Gandhi made it the symbol of political and economic self-rule.

More specifically, my concern in the analysis of commodities is in line with Nigel Thrift's emphasis on economies' generation of 'passionate interests'. Thrift, following Gabriel Tarde, argues, 'economies must be engaging: they must generate or scoop up affects and then aggregate and amplify them in order to produce value, and that must involve producing various mechanisms of fascination'.[32] One can see a similar set of processes at work in the affective life of khadi, for example. A simple piece of homemade cloth became an exemplary historic object through its association with, and manipulation by one of the most astute political leaders in history. Gandhian khadi thus became what Sherry Turkle calls an 'evocative object'.[33] Its power emerged and was sustained precisely through the cultivation of and attachment to affects such as national pride and belonging and economic self-sufficiency.

The 'evocative objects' of health and hygiene in colonial Bengal were mostly everyday things whose meaning, significance, and power shifted through history and in different social-economic-political domains. These objects and commodities, as I show in this book, signified the explicit medical and curative goal of cleansing, disinfecting, sanitizing, and purifying in the face of threat from contagions. They also represented anxieties about social, cultural, and moral contaminations that needed to be remedied. Contagion thus invoked the mode and pace by which sentiments and emotions became essential for creating the immense influence of these objects.

In bringing affect to bear upon the history of production and circulation of hygiene as a cultural project in late colonial Bengal, *Contagions of Feeling* seeks to provide a history of the present.[34] My book opens with recent debates in public health and draws attention to the affective charge that characterizes epistemologies and practices of public health and hygiene globally. Public health today, as it was during colonial times, is a set of bodily, cultural, and moral discourses that are prescriptions for individual and social health. In short, public health, as Deborah Lupton argues, is a 'socio-cultural product' and its specific forms change with shifts in social, cultural, and political contexts and desires.[35]

Contagions of Feeling is an interdisciplinary work. It draws from the field of affect studies and history of medicine to explore the crucial role of affect in getting ideas, practices, and objects – that constituted health and hygiene – moving and circulating in private and public spaces. Although for a long time hygiene has largely been the concern of historians, in recent years scholars from several other disciplines have analyzed hygiene, and this has also resulted in interdisciplinary perspectives. *Empires of Hygiene*, for example, is a compelling exploration of the deeply imperial constitution of hygiene. Priscilla Wald in *Contagious: Cultures, Carriers, and the Outbreak Narrative*, on the other hand, argues that outbreak narratives, far from becoming obsolete, are real and contemporary. *Contagions of Empire* contributes to this growing body of work by attending to the more routine elements of social, cultural, and political boundary-making that accompanied hygiene's everyday articulations. These ordinary and everyday articulations of hygiene were, nevertheless, extremely effective in constituting imperial, anti-colonial, and domestic orders of hierarchy and exclusion. *Contagions of Feeling* explores such articulations of hygiene in the context of late colonial Bengal by mapping the 'contact zones' where affect inhabited and suffused the texts and commodities of hygiene.[36]

Apart from the history and sociology of public health and medicine and affect studies, *Contagions of Feeling* also critically engages with the large body of studies of domesticity. Hygiene, both as an ideology and as a set of practices, defined the very core of domesticity. If domesticity was one of the most powerful cultural ideologies that re-wrote the script of modern social life, hygiene constituted one of its primary ordering mechanisms. Late nineteenth- and early twentieth-century Bengal, not unlike Judith Walsh's broader characterization of this era, represented an 'age of domesticity'.[37] Ideologies of nationalism and colonialism were intricately tied to discourses on health and wellbeing and the domestic became an important site on which these were being contested and reimagined. In colonial as well as nationalist ideologies, the imaginaries of nation, community, and family were distinctly gendered.

The relationship between domesticity, colonialism, and nationalism was forged on the backs of a gendered division of labor within the household. The 'women's question' consisted of a set of prescriptions that defined the values, duties, rights, and responsibilities of women inside and outside the middle class home. *Contagions of Feeling* focuses on advertisements for hygienic commodities and women's writings on the ethic of care in particular to highlight the gendered nature of ideologies and practices of hygiene in colonial Bengal. My goal, however, is not to point to an alternative genealogy of therapeutic-hygienic practices that was outside the purview of the colonial state and its institutional intermediaries. Rather, I argue that hygiene was a broad and multi-sited corporeal process that also included the Bengali middle class's attempts to write itself into history. In this process, middle class men, positioning themselves in relation to the colonial rule, laid claims to ordering the family and the household by drawing upon a number of conceptual, philosophical, and affective apparatuses.

Methods and sources

The origins of this book lie in my doctoral research. My dissertation was a historical–sociological analysis of the close link between hygiene and its most effective realm of persuasion and action – the household. While the history of hygiene and its coeval relationship with nation, domesticity, and culture remains the focus of this book, the analytical framework has shifted and the empirical material that I draw upon for that purpose has also changed. Specifically, in this book I explore the genealogy of hygiene by focusing on two entwined axes of articulation of hygienic practices and ideologies, namely affect and objects/commodities. Together they made hygiene meaningful and sensible as a social, cultural, and political practice and provided the material and cultural vocabulary of hygiene.

Hygiene did not simply represent the medical intervention of the colonial state, but was also a deeply cultural, political, and social project. The power of hygiene as a mechanism of cleanliness, order, and purification depended upon the degree to which it could affectively appropriate sites such as the household and the nation and thereby produce acceptable social practices from such appropriations. Such affective appropriations relied on transmissions of objects and commodities and their attendant ideologies not just in the official language, i.e. English, but also in the local language, Bengali. I have extensively examined the Bengali archives and translated archaic and modern Bengali writings to explore the cultural production of modern hygiene in colonial Bengal. I have been attentive to linguistic nuances of concepts and ideas about hygiene.

Contagions of Feeling, with a focus on colonial Bengal, utilizes data from a range of archival sources, including colonial public health records, monographs by colonial officials and administrators, English and Bengali newspapers, popular journals in Bengali, monographs on a variety of health and hygiene concerns in Bengali, and autobiographies of middle class Bengali women. The purpose of using the extensive archive of Bengali publications is not only to ensure richness of archival representation, but also to explore the expanse and depth of textual production on hygiene, sanitation, and health. I have also used information from two other popular cultural media – films and advertisements – in my study. Advertisements of the late nineteenth and early twentieth centuries constitute a rich archive of the moving history of commodities/products. They highlight the economic logics, political agendas, and affective tropes that produced hygiene in late colonial Bengal. I examine their affective articulations that 'moved' products such as soaps or patent medicines in and out of the marketplace, middle class homes, and the national space. The two films I analyze were produced much later than the other archival sources, in postcolonial India, and both of them retrospectively reflect upon the 1943 Bengal Famine and the massive annihilation of human lives that resulted from it. In that sense these films highlight the lingering affects of the history of health and hygiene in colonial India.

In the late nineteenth and the early twentieth centuries a thriving world of printing presses and publications became the primary medium for information exchange and knowledge production in colonial-urban Bengal. An active and politically engaged reading public already existed in urban Bengal during this period.[38] Bengal had witnessed the establishment of the first vernacular press in India and was the home of earliest indigenous printing and publishing industry. As Partha Chatterjee has rightly argued, it was through the 'production and circulation of printed texts that the discourses of modernity [were] disseminated in Bengal from the early nineteenth century'.[39]

By the second half of the nineteenth century, as small- and medium-scale Bengali entrepreneurs started investing in the growing market of books, newspapers, and periodicals, publishing became one of the largest and certainly most influential sectors of indigenous industry.[40] For example, in the short period of ten years between the 1857 Mutiny and 1867, the number of Bengali titles on sale rose from around 322 to over 900. There was an increase in the number of books that were published every year from around the 1850s. The massive growth in the production and circulation of books in Bengali was formidable enough to prompt the colonial government to put in place an administrative machinery for its surveillance.

My focus on Bengal is premised on the fact that at the end of the nineteenth and in the early twentieth centuries, Bengal still constituted, economically, the core of the British Empire in India (Calcutta was the capital of British colonial India until 1911). Moreover, the Bengali middle class was socio-culturally visible (even though its economic position was dwindling), because of its collaborative relations with the colonial administration and also because it led among the first articulate protests against British imperialism. Bengal was also important from the point of view of the growth of Western medical knowledge and institutions because it was here that the state support for medicine was first initiated.

Literature comprising of poetry, dramas, prose, and 'tales' constituted the largest percentage of Bengali publications. Titles in medicine were printed from around 1818 and their number steadily increased – from around 12 in 1818 to around 60 by the 1860s.[41] Between 1875 and 1896 the number of Bengali titles on science related topics was close to 800, of which around 600 were on medicine and health.[42] It is also worth noting that writings on health, apart from being published under the category of 'medicine', also spanned categories such as 'home science' and 'social issues'. Moreover, while in the early nineteenth century medical texts were simply translations or reprints of English texts, later, toward the end of the nineteenth and in the early twentieth centuries, medical writings were often original compositions. This transition marked a 'curious ambivalence' in the nationalist response toward pursuit of knowledge. On the one hand, it represented pragmatic appropriation of the new knowledge presented to Indians through colonial institutions, and on the other it reflected an insistence on the production of a 'distinctly Indian form of modern knowledge'.[43]

Wider debates over the representation and dissemination of knowledge and culture were thus evident in Bengali texts on health, hygiene, and medicine. According to some historians, it was this realignment and renegotiation that 'mediated a new discourse in the public domain that constituted our popular notion of science'.[44] It also led to enormous 'public' engagement in science and medicine in Bengali from the second half of the nineteenth century. A detailed survey of Bengali books, monographs, and periodicals on health, hygiene, and medicine is available in Benoybhushan Roy's (1995a) study *Uneesh Shatake Deshiya Bhashay Chikitsha Bigyan Charcha* (*The Pursuit of Medical Science in the Bengali Language in the Nineteenth Century*). Roy lists nearly 600 books and journals in Bengali on Western medicine, homeopathy, Ayurveda, *Unani*, and other Indian systems of medicine and therapeutics. The medical archive is situated within the above-discussed broader context.

In *Contagions of Feeling*, I have shifted from an exclusive focus on the mutual production of hygiene and domesticity to developing an understanding of hygiene and public health as a socio-cultural project. In an atmosphere of anti-colonial nationalism, such a project assumed added emphasis. Like its imperial counterpart, nationalism was equally a project of the physical, moral, and cultural disciplining of the individual and the collective. Public health in early twentieth-century colonial India was a patchwork of nineteenth-century public health diktats, driven by, on the one hand, a sanitarianism, which focused on the dangers of contamination of the environment by impurities in air and water. On the other hand, the early twentieth century marked the slow emergence of a model of public health where notions of individual responsibility and risk emerged as driving concerns. Infection and contagion had a strong hold on medical and lay imaginations at this time. Health and wellbeing were gradually defined as moral projects, wherein the policing and disciplining of individual and social bodies were paramount.[45]

Outline of chapters

Contagions of Feeling consists of an introductory chapter, four additional chapters and a conclusion. The Introduction lays out the analytical framework and archival focus of the book. It juxtaposes two moments in the history of hygiene and public health in India – the late colonial period, i.e. the late nineteenth and early twentieth centuries, and the present neoliberal time. I juxtapose these two moments in history to highlight the continued importance of affect, emotion, and feelings in charting trajectories of hygiene and public health. Of course, the ways in which affects have been made a part of discourses on health in these two historical periods are vastly different. In part, the economic and political incentives of these two moments make the respective trajectories of affect distinct. Nevertheless, in both these periods we see affect as the driving force behind the development of particular ideas and practices of hygiene. Moreover, in both periods affect is articulated through diverse texts on hygiene. In the context of colonial Bengal, on which I focus in the rest of the book, such texts include colonial health records, advertisements, and autobiographies, etc. Affective articulations, in fact, authorize and 'produce' the history of hygiene as a distinctly political discourse.

The second chapter, titled 'Alimentary Anxieties: Affect in Food and Hunger', examines the relationship between body, food, and nationalist imaginings. It explores the ways in which discourses on food, hunger, nutrition, diet, and sustenance supplied the ingredients for the imagining and disciplining of the 'body' of the nation and its citizens. Principally, it offers a critical reading of two modes of representation – Bengali monographs and periodicals on food, nutrition, and food adulteration, and two Bengali films, *Ashani Sanket* (Distant Thunder) and *Akaler Sandhaney* (In Search of Famine). It also explores the trope of hunger in Chittaprosad Bhattacharya's collection of paintings titled *Hungry Bengal* which present powerful images of death and devastation in the wake of the Bengal Famine.

'Gandhian Affects: Hygiene, Body, and *Swaraj*', the third chapter, explores the intimate links between Mahatma Gandhi's writings on sanitation, cleanliness, hygiene, *swadeshi*, and *satyagraha*. Bodily purity was one of the cornerstones of Gandhi's practice of political non-violence. Political self-rule as well as bodily sovereignty, for Gandhi, were ultimately moral issues. This chapter shows Gandhi's quest for the moral disciplining of the individual and political bodies, which brought together elements of hygiene, cleanliness, and moderation that were hierarchizing, and also contradictory. Specifically, I analyze the following writings of Gandhi: 'The Story of My Experiments with Truth', 'Key to Health', and 'Diet and Diet Reform', and articles from the *Indian Opinion* to bring to light his weaving together of values in hygiene and health with a particular caste and religious politics. In particular, I explore (a) his legal and social work in the context of a plague epidemic in South Africa and the plight of the

Indian community as a result of the aggressive plague control policies of the British government, and (b) his writings on what health meant to him and how modern medicine destroyed it.[46]

The fourth chapter – 'Imagining the Social Body: Competing Moralities of Care and Contagion' – explores autobiographical writings, short stories, non-fictional essays, and educational literature by middle class educated Bengalis on domesticity, cleanliness, and well-being. Through the analysis of these texts, this chapter maps the broader gender politics of care in late colonial Bengal. Analytically, this chapter is situated within a paradigm in feminist autobiographical criticism that calls for a 'post-colonial move', and examines autobiographical writings by previously colonized subjects in order to highlight interfaces of imperialism, patriarchy, religion, and class.

Chapter 5, titled 'Affective Remedies: Advertisements and Cultural Politics of Hygiene', explores the mutual production of empire, nation, domesticity, and consumption through the lens of commercial visual culture in late colonial Bengal. Through an analysis of advertisements for drugs, pills, and tonics from different therapeutic traditions, this chapter shows that medical marketing in colonial India consisted of several competing therapies, knowledge systems, and cultural repertoires. Allopathic, homeopathic, *hakimi*, and Ayurvedic remedies were equally highly in demand. These therapeutic systems together constituted a vibrant pluralism in the medical marketplace. The first half of the twentieth century witnessed a surge in advertisements for beauty products as well. Creams, soaps, and toiletries signaled a new phase in middle class consumption. These commodities were not simply products for material consumption, they also articulated hierarchical, albeit competing, perspectives on beauty, charm, and refinement. Since this time period was also politically vibrant, advertisements were often animatedly political in their tone, often drawing on tropes of empire and anti-colonialism. Advertisements for these commodities, as they attempted to create a new consumption class among women, were also, as I show, inherently gendered.

2
Alimentary Anxieties: Affect in Food and Hunger

This chapter explores the relationship between body, food, and nationalist imaginings. In particular, I investigate the question of what kinds of relationships were forged between an emergent nation and the people/bodies who constituted it (adequately fed, clothed, and sheltered) in early twentieth-century India's anti-colonial nationalist discourses. In other words, was there an analogy or correspondence between the making of the modern nation and making of the modern body, which could be identified with that national space? In what ways did food in particular (and related discourses about hunger, nutrition, diet, and sustenance) supply the ingredients that could offer a material body for the nation and a politico-moral-cultural body for the citizen? I focus on the paradoxes that were germane to the very imagination of the body that was attached to conceptions of the modern Indian nation by the early twentieth century.

Such paradoxes were intrinsic to the mutual imagining of the nation and its citizens. A postcolonial reading of the Indian nation's embodied history reveals that paradoxes were not recalcitrant. They rather constituted the social, cultural, and moral norms of the modern Indian nation. As I show elsewhere in the book, such paradoxes were in a sense indispensable to the modern, bourgeois Indian nationalist project. Although it is rarely if ever considered as such, one embodiment of hygiene in late colonial India was food. I define embodiment in this context as the set of processes through which ideas of modern hygiene were made literally and metaphorically the 'flesh' and material of the nation. Discourses on food, nutrition, and alimentation were therefore indispensable, and not only for conceptualizing how to feed a nation and its people. Food and palate were fundamental in configuring the nature of exchanges between the nation and its people, both during the late colonial moment in Bengal and India more generally and in postcolonial India.

I analyze writings in Bengali from monographs on food and nutrition, and from popular magazines on food, hygiene, and health. I also focus on two Bengali films which deal with the enduring anxieties surrounding the Bengal Famine, and more broadly the specter of hunger in postcolonial India. One of the films is by Satyajit Ray, *Ashani Sanket* (Distant Thunder), and the other is by Mrinal Sen, *Akaler Sandhaney* (In Search of Famine). Finally, this chapter examines Chittaprosad Bhattacharya's *Hungry Bengal*, a series of paintings and drawings documenting the human suffering of the Bengal Famine of 1943. The goal is to map some of the transference that took place with regard to anxieties around food, the body, survival, and/or wellbeing between the late colonial and postcolonial moments. This juxtaposition gives us an insight into the circulation of sentiments and affect that frames contemporary concerns with hunger and food insecurity.

The organic relationship between food, alimentation, and colonialism is now well documented, especially in the context of India. In literature and history especially, empire and food are explored in a mutual relationship of nurturing and dependence. Food has been analyzed as an optic through which related processes of capitalist appropriation of agricultural resources, different aspects of food production, distribution, and consumption, famine, emergence of new urban eating cultures and spaces, sanitary policing of marketplaces and food items, and the development of reading publics engaged in the cultivation of new culinary knowledge have been studied in ways that have revealed the varied and complex ways in which the empire was invested in matters of food, taste, and eating.

In what follows I investigate three aspects of the material, corporeal nation in the context of colonial Bengal and India more generally: (i) representations of the body that literally constituted the flesh and blood of the nation – its citizens; (ii) the 'processes' in and through which the nation became embodied in relation to food, its excess or absence, quality or quantity, and taste or need; and (iii) the paradox that organically and structurally marked the embodiment of the

Indian nation.[1] To analyze these aspects, I juxtapose two discursive registers in order to highlight the contrast between the two and also to be able to appreciate their uneasy co-existence in narratives of the nation. On the one hand are early twentieth-century debates on food adulteration, bodily maladies, and a broader rhetoric about social contamination. On the other hand I examine a contrasting set of discourses and representations of embodiment, nationhood, and food by focusing on the 1943 Bengal Famine. In the first section, titled 'Histories of food and the body', I explore some of the interdisciplinary debates that animate the scholarship on food, culture, and power reflecting on its analytical and empirical diversity.

The second section, called 'Food adulteration, embodiment, and the politics of anxiety', analyzes the trope of apprehension that was visible in most debates around food and the body in late colonial Bengal and India more broadly. The last section, called 'Famine's bodies', revisits the Bengal Famine centering on some of its representations that were produced in postcolonial India. As will have already been discussed, the shadow of drought, hunger, and food shortages persists despite 1943 being the last major famine in India. The main reason has remained the same – a highly inefficient supply chain. If not starvation, malnutrition is a critical issue facing large segments of poor rural and urban populations. Hunger continues to stir and move the public imagination in India today. Recent years have witnessed public memorialization of the 1943 famine through exhibitions and a variety of academic and journalistic writings.

The dynamic and historically contingent combination of food and hygiene is paramount, in short, to an understanding of an embodied history of the Indian nation. Apart from the conventional sense in which hygiene is understood, as a set of practices for the establishment and maintenance of health, I read hygiene also as a more extensive project of disciplining and normalizing the body politic and the social body. Both imperialism and nationalism were massive undertakings in lessons of hygiene and bodily management.[2] Articulated in a variety of discourses around diet, nourishment, and taste, food was creatively appropriated in cultural discourses around taste, economic discourses about production and poverty, and moral debates around self-control, indulgence, or dignity. Imaginations of the national body in relation to food and alimentation were framed in and marked by fissures and contradictions, of course. This fragile embodiment of the nation was contained in a body that was/is both present and absent at the same time.

Histories of food and the body

Historically, scholarship on food has been overwhelmingly anthropological. *The Eternal Food: Gastronomic Ideas and Experiences of Hindus and Buddhists* explores the dense hermeneutic world of Indian and Sri Lankan food, influenced heavily by religious principles of Hinduism and Buddhism.[3] While the religious and literary linkages are explored particularly in this book, the semiotics and semantics of food is worth noting. In the context of South Asia, Arjun Appadurai's 'semiotic virtuosity' is made possible by the power of food to create and distribute affect and 'strong emotion'.[4] In recent years food studies has become distinctly interdisciplinary. Underscoring the metaphor of travel and dispersion, in *Curried Cultures*, editors Krishnendu Ray and Tulasi Srinivas have analyzed the 'transnational' character of food and gastronomy in India. The move to study the transactional aspects of food through a variety of political and cultural aspirations signifies the turn toward locating and mapping the emotions, aspirations and affects that food produces and circulates.

This turn toward affect has been given a rich treatment by Parama Roy in her *Alimentary Tracts: Appetites, Aversions, and the Postcolonial* despite it being a thoroughly disciplinary text.[5] Through the analysis of food, and more importantly its affective accompaniments, Roy studies the production of the 'alimentary tract' as a 'boundary, a fiercely policed but also a contested and hotly trafficked one'. It is a border that for Roy was and has been pivotal in creating, debating, and sustaining certain thresholds of identity around questions of gender, caste, nationality, and class, among others. Roy's book offers a much-needed shift toward 'forms of embodiment' that accompanied colonial and nationalist projects. Unfortunately such projects were represented as disembodied histories of social, cultural, intellectual, and political contests, appropriations, and recoveries. *Alimentary Tracts* makes a productive use of both the representational and aesthetic, as well as material, aspects of this fundamental but overlooked concept of alimentation and its role in the life and afterlife of the Indian empire.

The history of Indian nationalism is replete with instances of the mediation of place by bodies creating meaningful histories of belonging and movement. For example, rice was an important ingredient in narratives of Bengali middle class identity in the mid nineteenth and early twentieth centuries. While rice was the staple food of Bengalis, during this time it gained a new purposeful symbolism when there was high incidence of Bengalis suffering from a range of digestive and gastrointestinal ailments. Numerous writings sought to explain the roots of this phenomenon along with possibilities for amelioration. These diseases were the result of bodies being unable to cope with the stresses of modern urban life, a hectic pace of work, and poor quality food. The quality of rice as a crucial part of Bengali fare was also threatened as a result of widespread food adulteration. Rice was being mixed with impurities so that it would look whiter. The culprits perpetuating such corruption were inevitably the traders and middlemen, who came from predominantly non-Bengali communities like the Marwaris or Biharis. Newspapers and popular journals were full of harsh criticisms for both these migrant communities and their unethical commercial practices. For a dyspeptic Bengali *babu* therefore, rice symbolized the flight from the lush Bengali countryside, fragrant rice fields, and good life to a wretched city existence that showed itself on the wasted bodies of the *bhadralok*. The urban jungle of Calcutta and rice came together in this curious way to create a particular identity for the physically and culturally emaciated Bengali *babu*.

Food adulteration, embodiment, and the politics of anxiety

In times of famine and food shortage of the kind brought on, if not guaranteed, by the exigencies of imperial rule, anxiety as an affective trope emerged with regard to the disintegration of the Bengali body from consumption of impure and adulterated food items. In this affective framework, the Bengali body was on the threshold of complete ruin. Economic mismanagement by dubious social agents had perpetuated a state where the quality of food had deteriorated – the result of being mixed with impure substances. Essential fare like rice and milk were the most notable adulterated ingredients of daily consumption. While the resultant slow degeneration toward death was almost imperceptible, it nonetheless produced a body that was at the same time an object, a metaphor, and a signifying medium in the late colonial context.

Epidemics and famines bring out a corporeal history of colonial India that was glaring, wretched, and heartbreaking. Much has been written on the visual nature of famines in India. The Bengal Famine of 1943, for example, was an episode in Indian history that led to the publication of a wide range of texts, from novels, films, photographs, reports, and journalistic essays to academic writings that significantly contributed to the creation of a cultural space. The recent publication of Madhusree Mukherjee's *Churchill's Dirty War: The British Empire and the Ravaging of India During World War II* (2011) is a contribution to the archive on the devastations that the Bengal Famine unleashed, clothed in complex imperial politics. Coincidentally, 2011 was also the year that Chittaprosad Bhattacharya's sketches of the Bengal Famine went on display at the Delhi Art Gallery.[6] Such visual chronicles of this famine have in recent years re-created an embodied haunting of India by its colonial past that finds strange resonance in today's postcolonial neoliberal world, characterized by poverty, food shortages, and regional famines.[7] The history of colonial India is replete with representations of epidemic diseases, like cholera and plague, that killed thousands.

Representations of epidemics were unlike those of famines. The agony and affliction that was portrayed in the diseased or deceased patients of cholera or plague was not as brazen as for bodies affected by famine – dead or alive. In fact the distinction between life and death for famine victims was often blurred. Suzanne Hatty talks about bodies affected by epidemics as 'disordered bodies' that significantly influenced conceptions of bodies in Medieval Europe.[8] Representations of epidemics in colonial India signified 'disorder' with connotations of contagion breaking boundaries of class, caste, and gender. In contrast, images of famine were much more 'stereotypical' in their depictions of starved bodies reduced to merely skin and bones.[9]

Epidemics were typically represented through a number of depictions. Dead bodies shrouded in white sheets; mass migrations of people; bodies being carried on carts; vaccination campaigns; and images of fumigation during plague epidemics (Hatty, 1999). As Roger Cooter argues persuasively in his essay on public health posters during the HIV/AIDS epidemic, the visual media of epidemics in early twentieth-century India operated by 'evoking a controlled form of fear and anxiety for purposes of rational governance over personal and/or national life'.[10] In literature, epidemics like cholera, plague, and malaria have been woven into narratives around science and medicine, colonial trade and travels, and the lives of English men and women and their exchanges with and involvement in the lives of the colonized, and used as tropes of poverty and suffering in rural India.[11]

While the embodiment of epidemics and famines was prominent in the visual and non-visual, literary and non-literary print world, such representations were fewer and far between when it came to food adulteration. Yet food adulteration was an issue that caused much concern among public health authorities and a section of the educated public, to the extent that much was written about it in the popular press of the time. Food adulteration was a complex issue to tackle and resolve given that most of the time it was hard to detect such practices. Evaluating food adulteration was often a time-consuming and expensive process on the part of the colonial state. Kavita Ray offers a detailed history of food adulteration and some of the ameliorative strategies undertaken by the British government in Bengal, for example.[12] She has argued that despite the colonial government sanctioning crucial pieces of legislation to curb it, instances of food adulteration remained rampant and mired in complicated local politics.[13]

The Bengal Municipal Act of 1884, the Municipal Amendment Act of 1917, and finally the Bengal Food Adulteration Act of 1919 were the last in a series of acts that tried to check food adulteration in Bengal. The 1919 Act provided for the 'prohibition of sale etc., of food, not of the proper nature or substance or quality, prohibition of sale etc., of articles of food which were not of the prescribed standard or purity'.[14] It also made illegal the storage of any adulterant in production or processing sites for 'ghee [clarified butter], wheat flour, etc'. This act was finally able to bring both urban and rural Bengal under one purview as far as monitoring food adulteration was concerned. Newspapers, popular journals, and advertisements were abuzz with strong condemnation of food adulteration and its impact on the health and wellbeing of the people of Bengal. The commonest items of adulteration were milk, ghee, mustard oil, and wheat flour, each of which had its own particular economic, social, and cultural significance, which led to each of these commodities developing a unique history as the target of anti-adulteration measures and public critique. Anne Hardgrove offers a fascinating analysis of how ghee (clarified butter), for example, played an important role in the history of the Marwaris as a 'political constituency' under British rule in Calcutta.[15] And rice, for example, became a commodity that attained a heightened cultural and social significance in late colonial India in discourses on poverty, nutrition, diet, and national belonging.[16]

The concerns about food adulteration took shape in a distinct set of discourses depending upon who the affected public was. So for example, as mentioned above, for the educated Bengali middle class debates about food adulteration were crucially about health, vitality, class and caste distinctions, and formation of a cultural self. For the colonial state, it was about public health governance and imperial identity. In *Tea and Food Adulteration, 1834–75*, Judith Fisher writes about the history of tea adulteration and lays bare a complex imperial genealogy, though at a different historical moment. She argues:

> [T]he importance of tea as a healthful, particularly, British drink made the adulteration of the beverage a significant matter for social and moral concern. Adulterated tea was primarily from China and so was typed 'foreign' and unclean in contrast to tea imported from Assam, India that was defined as 'British' and healthy.[17]

Embodiment in the context of food adulteration involves analysis of the ways in which food adulteration and its significance (physical and moral) were introduced and became part of social, cultural, and political discourses of that period. It means tracing in particular how certain ideas, values, and commodities became part and parcel of a broader public culture and affect. In my article on the cultural politics of taste, I dwelt on the role that rice played in cementing a sense of Bengali self-identity. Rice and milk were two fundamental items in the gastronomical ensemble that made up discourses on food in late colonial Bengal. A fulfilling and nutritious conception of a meal included rice as well as other items prepared at home. Rice was made important at the interface of ideas of nutrition on the one hand, and an allegiance to the existing gastronomic tradition on the other.

The importance of rice lay not only in its being the staple food but also in its being a response to a number of socio-economic and political processes, which were specific to colonial Bengal. It became a symbol of resistance to the 'colonization of taste' as C.A. Bayly talks about with reference to cloth and its connection to the genealogy of twentieth-century *swadeshi*.[18] In late colonial Bengali middle class discourses on food, rice also became meaningful and desirable in its opposition to wheat. In the Bengali *bhadralok* discourses wheat became a synecdoche for a number of non-Bengali communities. These communities, who based their diet on roti (bread) made from wheat and daal (lentils), were pejoratively labeled as Hindustanis. Therefore, rice became an index of othering that had external (colonial) as well as internal Indian referents.[19] I cite a few examples of such concern that were seen often in monographs and magazine essays. In an article titled 'Swasthya Samashya' (The Problem of Health), the author stressed,

> For us, the most fundamental items of food are rice and milk. In recent times their high prices have forced people to the verge of chronic starvation. In the name of free trade and commerce, we are exporting rice every year, worth ten crores of rupees – is not it the reason for high prices of food like rice?[20]

Similarly, in a book titled *Bangalir Khadya O Pushti* (1935), author Nibaran Chandra Bhattacharya wrote,

> A strong opposition has developed against the most vital food of the Bengalis–rice. We have been ordered to give up easily available, moderately priced rice, which our own country produces and instead survive on flour imported from foreign countries.[21]

The Bengali middle class was actively involved in the cause of prevention and control of food adulteration. Many were physicians, public health professionals, and educationists – Sundari Mohan Das, Chunilal Basu, Indubhushan Sen, P.C. Ray, Chandra Nath Basu, Aswinikumar Biswas, Gyanendra Saha, Srishchandra Goswami, Nagendra Chandra, and Rajarshi Dasgupta.[22] They frequently wrote for Bengali popular journals and authored topic-based monographs. Titles included *Khadya* (Food), *Anyasamasya* (Scarcity of Rice/Food), *Bangalir Khadya Samasya* (Bengalis and Their Food Scarcity), *Bangalir Khadya* (The Food of Bengalis), and *Khadya Tattwa* (Treatise on Food), to give a few examples.

There was a lively set of debates that were framed around the food crisis, the lack of nutritious and pure food, adulteration, and diet. Ideas and affects that were commonly evoked were those of the nation (*desh*), society (*samaj*), community (*jati*), and family (*paribar*). Food adulteration was couched in qualities of strength, resilience, health, and purity. For example, Bhudeb Mukhopadhyay argued either for a strictly vegetarian diet, one that the 'Aryans' had, or one that involved moderate consumption of meat, the way the 'Germans' or the 'French' did.[23] Masculinity was another key concern that was intricately tied to the notion of strength and toughness and that finally came from nutritious and pure food capable of re-invigorating both body and spirit. Therefore, certain food items were highly debatable commodities especially when it came to their suitability for the health of Bengalis. Meat (especially beef), bread, sugar, and milk became topics on both sides of the debate. Some felt that milk was in fact a highly beneficial item of consumption, or for example that a fully vegetarian diet was the reason behind lean and feeble Bengali constitutions because it lacked protein-rich foods.

Adulteration came in the way of procuring and consuming good quality food. As Utsa Ray points out, 'the arguments on nutrition became inextricably conjoined with arguments on "pure" food in the past and "adulterated" food in the present. Pure had a double meaning. On the one hand, purity represented a critique of colonial administration and forced the latter to impose more stringent policies in relation to adulteration. On the other hand, purity also signified food that was untouched, which could imply the British as well as those unnamed people (ranging from cultivators to cooks and sweetmeat makers) who were involved in the making and handling of food items, which the middle class Bengali was obliged to consume. The present signified 'new' and 'foreign' for the Bengali middle class. These two meanings together constituted the discourse of nutrition in colonial Bengal. The colonial state's economic policies had to take these cultural meanings into account when dealing with the question of adulteration'.[24]

Anxiety provided a decisive ground on which woes and disquiet about food adulteration helped in the manufacture of social, cultural, and moral communities. It linked the domain of bodies (the Bengali body and the national body) to that of a regional (Bengali) and national affect. Nation became linked to the material world of commodities (which signified food adulteration or the possibility of food adulteration) and that of bodies (diseased and dyspeptic) through a deeply felt distress and uncertainty. Commodities like rice, ghee, mustard oil, and milk therefore became animated with questions of purity, contamination, and health. These food items became nodal points for the emergence and consolidation of discourses on colonialism, nationalism, productivity, self-subsistence, diet, and nourishment. Food adulteration was invisible, unlike the starkness of famine-ravaged bodies in the context of colonial India. Yet it became a concrete and affective terrain on which crucial questions around consumption and health were debated to the extent that food adulteration became synonymous with anxieties about the body, community, and nation.[25]

Famine's bodies

The year 2013 marked the seventieth anniversary of the Bengal Famine. Exhibitions and panel discussions commemorated 'the things we forgot to remember'.[26] In 2011 Chittaprosad Bhattacharya's sketches from his acclaimed work *Hungry Bengal* were put on display at the Delhi Art Gallery.[27] Somnath Hore's works on the 1943 famine were also exhibited in 2013. What Stuart McLean has aptly called the 'publicly enacted signifiers of social memory' have revisited the immense horror and suffering of that time in order to reiterate its importance as a moment that altered the history of modern India.[28] There has been a slew of academic writings also, critically reviewing the significance of the Bengal Famine of 1943 from both historiographical and literary perspectives. It is contended that the Bengal Famine has often been forgotten because of its close temporal contiguity to World War II, India's independence, and the Partition, and many recent events of remembrance of the famine have been framed around this omission.

David Arnold stresses the importance of understanding famines as more than critical antecedents to present experiences of large-scale food shortages and starvation. He reinforces their centrality to the 'new social history' lens to scrutinize the interlinked networks of food, power, and culture at moments when economic and social resources had been completely exhausted. Arnold's influential work on famines has filled a void in history scholarship on famines, especially their significance for social history.[29] Famines in India, including the Bengal Famine of 1943, have been studied predominantly by economists trying to study what 'caused' them. Historians and especially social historians therefore brought about a whole new way of studying famines by scrutinizing what these massive processes of death and migration meant for the complex grids of peoples' everyday lives, especially those lives that were hit the hardest by acute food shortages. Cultural and literary representations of the famine have provided another set of powerful narratives, which have focused on the meaning of the famine as it unfolded in and through the daily lives of ordinary people. The Bengal Famine has been depicted not only as a tale of death and suffering but also as a struggle against the injustices of those in power against those who lacked it.

Narratives and representations of the Bengal Famine, like other famines both in India and globally, have summoned an important question, that of chronology – the beginning and end of a famine. Christopher Morash asks a provocative question about the Irish Famine of 1846. 'So when was the Famine?' he asks. He goes on to say, 'The problem of assigning it a date is not the same as that which pertains to historical events of the distant past, where we know that a queen was born, or campaign fought, or a pharaoh entombed, but we are not quite sure when.'

In the case of the famine, it is the event itself which eludes definition. There is no single, clear consensus as to what constituted the famine'.[30] In the literature on the 1943 Bengal Famine there is a similar concern that has become integral to an understanding of the magnitude of the event in all its spread and complexity. Despite being called the Famine of 1943, the validity of this date as marking a clear-cut beginning and end has been questioned, given that starvation and the resultant deaths occurred over a protracted period of time. Paul Greenough puts it aptly,

> The calamitous months of 1943–44 were only the most intense phase of a decades-long period of food scarcity and rural distress in Bengal. A demonstrable decline in rice consumption since the end of the nineteenth century, plus a rapid increase in this century of undesirable alternatives to tenancy, such as sharecropping and agricultural wage-labor, make it at least arguable that hunger and economic insecurity have been the lot of millions of Bengalis for more than eighty years.[31]

And it has remained a powerful pneumonic in the collective memory of Bengal because of its magnitude and severity.

> Like the memory of the great depression in the industrialized world, the famine is regularly harked back to by thoughtful Bengalis and continues to have an impact on consciousness. When a decennial census-taker wants to determine the approximate date of some vital event in the Bengali villager's life, one means he has at hand is to ask whether the event was before or after the famine. This is because *pancaser manvantar* or the 'famine of fifty' was a calamity no Bengali of the older generation can forget. According to my estimate its toll was around 3.5 million lives. Further, it was a cause of impoverishment for millions of others, who dispossessed themselves in order to purchase food. Whether considered demographically or economically, the famine was on a par with the two other most disruptive events in twentieth-century Bengal – the partition-migration of 1947 and the 1971 war for the liberation of Bangladesh from Pakistan.[32]

Despite difficulties around assigning a clear-cut date as to the start and end of the famine, 1943–1944 marked an abysmal peak in large-scale migration and deaths in Bengal. In a similar vein Margaret Kelleher designates the 1943 famine as one that was 'catastrophic in its effects' and 'as a living memory for many Bengalis, the "famine of fifty" remains a measure of time and change'.[33]

The archive on the 1943 famine is a collage of different kinds of texts – novels, short stories, and drama. The visual chronicles consist of films, photographs, ink sketches, linocut sketches, and paintings. Significantly, the hungry body was not the province of any one representational technique; diverse media collectively summoned the bodies and the affects of the famine. Multiple visual representations powerfully created the Bengal Famine as a social, economic, and moral emergency. In both their content and form, they produced the famine as an embodied and affective event.[34] In other words, these media created a cultural, moral, and political community around an event that was rendered unreadable given the intensity and enormity of the catastrophe.[35]

In this chapter, the two films that I discuss are *Ashani Sanket* (Distant Thunder, 1973), a film by Satyajit Ray, and *Akaler Sandhaney* (In Search of Famine, 1980), a film by Mrinal Sen. *Ashani Sanket* is the story of a village as its people suffer through the economic woes created by WWII that signal the famine of 1943–1944. The film is centered on an educated Brahmin, Gangacharan, who earns his livelihood by teaching the village children and performing religious rites for villagers. He is respected for his education and wisdom (which is connected to his upper caste status of course), and despite being of moderate means, he is very conscious of the status he enjoys for being a well-read caste Brahmin. He is a mean-minded and crafty man given to maneuvering situations to his own advantage. For example, he tries to be consciously indifferent to and dismissive of the plight of a poor man who has a large and hungry family and almost nothing to feed them and who in desperation asks for help from Gangacharan. Gangacharan's wife Ananga, on the other hand, is a kind young woman who assures her husband that if need be she will go out to work with other women of the village, which to Gangacharan is unacceptable.

The war ravages on and dries up the rice supply of the village, and the film shows how one by one the villagers and their families are hit by the assault of food shortage. Warplanes in the sky portend frightful times to come and on the ground slowly terrifying scenes of hunger and starvation unfold. Men take dire steps to feed their families. Chutki, a married woman and a friend of Ananga's, runs away to the city with a man she dreaded because she is not able to endure the pain of hunger. The situation in the village worsens fast as rice becomes almost impossible to procure and there are instances of civic disorder at the house of the village *jotdar* as he refuses to sell any more rice. Gangacharan's pride in himself is thoroughly shaken and at the end of the film one sees him a humbled man who shows signs of some compassion as he completes the funeral rites of a low caste, untouchable woman lying dead at the boundary of the village. As the family members of an elderly man who is unable to provide for his family anymore walk toward Gangacharan's house in search of some food, Ananga asks her husband for a solution, to which Gangacharan says that instead of two they will try to provide for ten. The film ends with silhouettes of hundreds of villagers walking slowly toward the city with their families in a long line, leaving the village in search of food.

Mrinal Sen's *Akaler Sandhaney* is the story of a film crew from Calcutta in its quest to make a film on the Bengal Famine of 1943.

It centers on the film crew's excursion to a village and the ordeals it faces there, while shooting for the film. The villagers are excited at the arrival of the crew as it marks a break from their daily lives of poverty and drudgery. The film focuses on a few characters from the village as the stories of their lives take shape around the activities of the film crew. All is well until one of the actresses leaves the film because of a temper tantrum and the director of the film is at a loss about the completion of the project. The rest of the film delves into apprehensions of and confrontations between the villagers (as they try to deal with their memories and fears of the famine and the fragility of their lives and values) and the film crew, its urban middle class sensibilities and inability to appreciate and understand some of the fears which the villagers dwell in.

Both *Ashani Sanket* and *Akaler Sandhaney* are framed outside the immediate time frame of the famine. They are not about the experiences of people during the time of the famine *per se*. Yet both films narrate the famine in interesting ways – *Ashani Sanket* forecasts the coming of the famine, and *Akaler Sandhaney* takes a look back at it. *Sanket* means sign and *Ashani* is thunder. *Ashani Sanket* centers on everyday (therefore indistinct) developments in the village just before starvation, death, and migration assumed catastrophic proportions. Yet the film precisely focuses on those daily occurrences which, while invisible, are the tell tale signs of a mammoth tragedy in the making. The famine was after all a man-made disaster that was the result of a reckless and brutal set of economic policies that were brought together by the colonial government and other economic and political actors wielding power and influence that ultimately crushed the poor. In *Akaler Sandhaney* we visit a village in Bengal three decades after the famine took place, yet the famine for many villagers is not over. Deprivation and poverty continue unabated in their lives, though it remains hidden from the view of privileged city folks. The famine thus continues to frazzle the bodies of the already vulnerable.

Both films are then about the ominous signs either of a time that culminated in the famine in *Ashani Sanket*, or a time that happens a long 30 years after the famine in *Akaler Sandhaney*. Both anticipate and recount the everyday and sometimes hidden horrors and pains of poverty-related deprivation, which characterize the lives of the poor and under-privileged. The callousness, depravity, and indifference which the privileged and powerful have unleashed on the vulnerable is a never-ending reality. The everyday ordeals of common people, and their struggle to procure the basic ingredients for survival – physical, social, and moral – are always present as signs of an impending disaster or traces of its aftermath. It is in their perpetuity that the famine continues. Both films (since they are set preceding the famine and following the famine) paint rural Bengal in images that might not be as calamitous as if they were set during the famine itself, but are nonetheless harsh and precipitous. Hunger, disease, and death therefore remain the violent yet unavoidable underside of the relationship that is forged between food, survival, and the modern Indian nation. The pain of hunger and death on the one hand deny the physical and material continuation of the body. Yet the same bodies in their hunger, decay, and death reiterate the deeply corporeal nature of affective communities that form around food, alimentation, and nationhood.

Neither of the films portrays starving or dying bodies, which were otherwise typical images of the Bengal Famine represented in paintings, drawings, and sketches. The depiction of corpses lying around, being devoured by dogs or vultures, has been recurrent in the archive on the Bengal Famine. Rather, in the films death is either represented as a portent, revealed in the quiet starvations in the village and the first food riot at the *jotdar*'s granary, or in the indifference of the film crew members, who in their gallant desire to revisit the Bengal Famine are simply oblivious to the hunger and starvation that imperil the villagers' meager everyday lives.

In contrast to these two well-known films on the Bengal Famine, the works of artists such as Chittaprosad Bhattacharya and Somnath Hore represent the horrors of mass hunger, migration, and death in a starkly different way. Chittaprosad Bhattacharya has been viewed as one of the most politically minded artists of modern India. A Communist Party card holder member, Chittaprosad's art was steeped in his political commitments, or in other words, his art could not be thought of as separate from his politics. In recent years, there has been much interest in Chittaprosad's work, both in the art world and in academia. In 2011, the Delhi Art Gallery displayed his artwork and memorabilia.

Besides his drawings, watercolor paintings and prints, the exhibition at the Delhi Art Gallery included Chittaprosad's published writings, letters, posters, photographs, and puppets. For the show, the gallery also published four lavishly produced books that charted the artist's life, work, and thoughts. One of these volumes consists of the facsimile edition of his book *Hungry Bengal*, all copies of which were seized and burnt by the British. A single copy had survived in a bank vault in Calcutta.[36,37] One of the most acclaimed works of the artist, *Hungry Bengal* is a set of 22 black and white sketches, which appeared serially in the Communist journal, *People's War*, when the artist toured the famine hit districts of Bengal in 1943–1944 and later.

Hungry Bengal is a hard-hitting portrayal of the destruction that the Bengal Famine brought in its wake, which was unparalleled in its scale and immensity. A chronicle of the human cost of the famine through a set of stark sketches and commentary, it remains one of the most invaluable archives of the Bengal Famine today. Chittaprosad's style has been linked to the artistic conventions which marked the works of artists with strong communist commitments. In analyzing his work and his style, political historian Rajarshi Dasgupta argues,

> From the 1940s, Chittaprosad started working for the 'CPI's publications and propaganda. The next few years witnessed a formidable range of artworks, marked by strikingly original pictorial language, spanning wide thematic and technical variations. Cartoons, illustrations, posters, prints, portraits of national and international communist leaders, pictorial commentaries of radical movements, documentary images and texts, new calligraphies, graphic improvisations – everything in keeping with the constraints and needs of the medium suitable to communist propaganda'.[38]

As Dasgupta argues, the Bengal Famine provided an immediate reason behind a surge of socially conscious artistic production. As he writes, a large number of artists felt compelled to address the reality of famine at this critical juncture, and held exhibitions with works that pointedly engaged with the context.[39] Chittaprosad, Zainul Abedin, Gobardhan Ash, and Somnath Hore were artists of the time who were deeply involved in representing some of the horrors of the Bengal Famine. But as Dasgupta says,

> [u]nlike the others, the work of these artists essentially had little to do with the available artistic conventions or established

aesthetic concerns. Rather than achieving the status of works of immense beauty and appeal that addressed suffering their works were more like prosaic headlines, news bulletins and eyewitness reports – practical documents that accurately recorded the truth about the famine, without any frills. In other words, what they tried was precisely to subordinate art, as an elite practice, to a political labour of representation tested on the ground of objective reality, in the manner of someone reporting from a field of destruction in a clinical spirit.[40]

Hungry Bengal narrates the abject suffering of the poor people of Bengal whose lives were completely decimated by the famine of 1943–1944. All of his sketches, paintings, and linocuts in this series focus on women, men, and children lying around in their homes starved and dying, reduced to bare bones – signs of wretchedness everywhere. For example, in *Hungry Bengal* the subjects are a mother holding her naked child, a man sitting under a tree holding an empty earthen pot, a broken hut, and two bodies lying on the ground dead or about to die. Another of his sketches depicts a dead body surrounded by vultures ready to feast on it. One of the legs of the corpse has already been eaten while a dog looks on hungrily is better. There are a couple of his works in this series, which depict an old man lying either in a relief camp or a hospital on the brink of death, reduced to just a skeletal frame.

Dasgupta argues that these sketches, paintings, and linocuts are examples of the 'socialist realism' that emerged in the wake of the Soviet Exhibition of 1932 – a surge of 'aesthetic experiments that gave new energies as well as languages to nascent communist movements in colonized countries'.[41] True to this tradition, Chittaprosad's pieces from *Hungry Bengal* tried to voice the suffering of the people of Bengal with an economy of artistic representation that was effected by the use of particular techniques that gave a distinct effect. The thin lines and dark thick strokes were used to great effect in *Hungry Bengal*, for instance in his portrayal of two bodies lying on the mud floor of a hut, one face down and one face up, while the thatched roof lies collapsed in the background, pieces of broken pots and pans strewn around underlining the grimness of the situation. This particular sketch points to the utter desperation which forced millions to leave their village homes for the city where lay their last hopes of getting food.

There is another sketch in this series, which portrays a few huts of an abandoned village, all of whose inhabitants have fled to the city in search of food. A man sick and exhausted lies in a relief camp cot, his exposed bones showing the hollow starved state he is in. Jutting out from his torso are two bare legs, which look more like posts than human limbs. The stomach of the sick man is shown as a crater in a frame of bones held together by a thin sheet of skin. The sparse surrounding closely resembles the slender frame of the man and the severity of suffering that the man represents in this sketch. Another striking sketch is that of a mother holding her unclothed child in her arms, an empty earthen pot by her side. The poignancy of this piece is evident in the pose of the child, hanging his or her head, and the mother's face which is shaded in black, illustrating the helplessness of the mother unable to provide food for her child. Yet despite such helplessness, there is still a sliver of hope that seems to seep out of this image.

Many of the paintings, sketches, and linocuts represent objects like pots and pans that are symbolic of food and hearth and are seen lying empty or broken right beside the starved and dying subjects of the famine that Chittaprosad chronicled. A ubiquitous sign of cooking and food, these earthen pots symbolize their dire absence. The hunger of starved women, men, and children gets heightened as these empty containers point to a bleak present and more ominously a terrible future. The entanglement of human bodies and material objects of everyday use in domestic spaces highlights powerfully what was destroyed most enormously and utterly in the wake of the Bengal Famine – family lives, homes, and households. It is the paradox of materiality represented in these images, which is affirmed (food and the physicality of human bodies in distress) and denied (empty earthen pots, broken huts, and dying or dead bodies) at the same time, that creates a deep affect around food, metabolism, vitality, and life. Postcolonial histories of food and culture will be haunted by the Bengal Famine – a terrible and callous failure of the British state and its subsidiaries, leading to the huge exodus of starving millions to the city, and their failure to reach the destination. We see such affect at work in the sixtieth anniversary commemoration of the Bengal Famine or the publication of scholarly works on artists like Chittaprosad.

James Vernon in his book, *Hunger: A Modern History*, argues that the history of hunger is indeed a modern and imperial one. Famines and hunger in Ireland and India contributed profoundly to a sensibility where the hungry and starving became moral symbols of the failure of states and societies to feed human beings. In recent years the Bengal Famine of 1943 has resurged in public memory. Exhibitions, interviews, and books have attempted to retrieve some of the horror and pain of mass starvation and deaths that decimated rural and urban Bengal. These public commemorations become affective transits between the past and the future. The shadows of famine's destruction have not left us. This chapter analyzes how affect made food a constant object of anxiety and distress in colonial and postcolonial India. I offer readings of two registers of this affect – the Bengal Famine in artistic and cultural representations, and the persistent unease and consternation around food adulteration that were evoked in late colonial discourses in Bengal and that continue to be evoked in postcolonial India.[42]

3
Body, Hygiene, and the Affective Politics of Gandhi's *Swaraj*

'I had been used to fasting, now and again, but for purely health reasons.' Fasting, however, had much deeper implications for Mahatma Gandhi. In 1925, when he wrote the above words, Gandhi was discussing his experiment in using fasting as a 'technology of self' (*The Story of My Experiments with Truth*, 1925). 'That fasting was necessary for self-restraint,' he added. 'I learnt from a friend.' Nearly 25 years later, he was far more categorical: 'Control of the palate is the first essential in the observance of the vow. I saw that complete control of the palate made the observance very easy and so I now pursued my dietetic experiments not merely from the vegetarian's but also from the *brahmachari*'s point of view' (*Diet and Diet Reform*, 1949).

If there was one concern that formed the basis for Gandhi's moral, spiritual, and political journey, it was the centrality of his engagements with the body and its potential to contribute to national self-rule or *swaraj*. Indeed, as Joseph Alter argues, 'Gandhi's search for Truth was manifest in his biomoral politics and that his experimentation with vegetarianism, diet reform, nature, cure, and *brahmacharya* must be understood as integral to his project of *satyagraha* as a whole' (Alter, 2000a, 200b). One of Gandhi's major texts, *Key to Health*, is a guidebook in which he laid down what he called the 'rules' of health. One of his most popular writings, *Key to Health* is a compendium of a variety of food items and the elements of the natural environment, which contribute in a major way to the maintenance of the body. His *The Story of My Experiments with Truth* is similarly a narrative that chronicles Gandhi's bodily physiological experiments as he performed frequent fasts, tried various diets, and practiced sexual abstinence.

These biomoral exercises were to his mind the indispensable steps to India's political self-rule or *swaraj*. This chapter explores some of the practices that Gandhi regularly experimented with and from time to time made public as moral and political prescriptions for the nation. Not only in his pivotal writings like *Key to Health* but also within the rest of his large oeuvre of work, his engagement with the body and bodily practices remained a central issue. Gandhi's political goals were inseparable from corporeal practices. As Joseph Alter put it,

> I am convinced that what Gandhi said and did with regard to sex, food, and nature cure entails a reevaluation of who he was and what his place in Indian history should be. The simple point is that by starting with the body one is better able to make sense of the Mahatma in particular and important features of the nationalist project as a whole.[1]

So an engagement with Gandhi's nationalist politics remains incomplete if one does not attend to his bodily and biomoral experiments.[2] In this chapter, I analyze his writings on fasts, sanitation, and medicine. I also explore the affective politics of Gandhi's biomoral endeavors.

The Story of My Experiments with Truth chronicles what Gandhi considered to be the significant moments of his life in terms of his spiritual, moral, and political life, from his childhood, friendships, and travel to South Africa, to his years in India as one of the foremost leaders of anti-colonial nationalist politics, and is a window to his affective and emotional life as well. By affective I mean the pleasures, frustrations, woes, and confusions that expressed some of Gandhi's inner sensibilities during the course of his life-journey. Such affective densities give a distinct texture to him as a moral and ethical being affected by the vicissitudes of life, willingly or otherwise. Exploring his affective life becomes doubly meaningful because self-manipulation of affect was a crucial dimension in Gandhi's broader politico-moral project. Gandhi's writings are replete with practices, the explicit goals of which were to discipline and restrain 'passions' or affects, which he deemed opposite to the very spirit of his theory of political self-rule. Denial, pain, suffering, grief, and moving beyond were precisely the crux of his spiritual and moral experiments. This chapter is a scrutiny of Gandhi's biomoral and affective politics that formed the backbone of his notion of *swaraj*.[3]

For this chapter I analyze Gandhi's writings and reflections on the body, health, diet, and medicine in *The Story of My Experiments with Truth, Diet and Diet Reform, Key to Health, Hind Swaraj*, and articles in the *Indian Opinion*. The goal is to explore the intertwining of his corporeal and affective lives as a roadmap to his political aspirations. For example, at the same time as experimenting with vegetarian, uncooked, or milk-free diets, doing relief work in the event of a plague outbreak, or undertaking a fast, Gandhi wrote down his affective fluctuations as well. To my mind it is important that we read both registers in a parallel manner, given that controlling particular affects and fostering their opposites was at the heart of Gandhi's lifelong political work.

I raise the following questions in this chapter: (1) how and in what ways did affect play a cardinal role in Gandhi's moral and political *swaraj*?; (2) how did his experiments in diet, fasts, and sanitation throw into relief his trials with diverse affects?; and (3) in what ways did notions of contagion (bodily, social, and moral) play out in Gandhi's *swaraj*?

The chapter is divided into four main sections. In the first section, entitled 'Body, affect, and Gandhi', I locate my arguments within the current scholarship on Gandhi, especially where this recasts his politico-moral projects, moving away from a limited binary (saint versus crafty political leader) concept to a more nuanced understanding of his personhood. The second section is called 'Gandhi's fasts', and it studies the recurrent fasts that Gandhi undertook and how those trials were intimately connected to his experiments with emotions and their control. The third section, 'Race and Gandhi's politics of hygiene', is a commentary on Gandhi's ideas about hygiene, sanitation, and cleanliness, and the relationship he conceptualized between his own body and that of the body politic. In the final section, 'Medicine as contagion', I explore some of his writings on medicine and his categorical unwillingness to give any credit to medicine as having the ability to truly cure disease.

At the outset, I would like to comment on the nature of my engagement with Gandhi's life and politics in this chapter. While it is located within the events of his life and work, this chapter in no way follows a strict chronological narrative. I explore Gandhi's politics of the body, self, and nation from a historical-sociological perspective while at the same time locating myself in some of the contemporary and interdisciplinary research on Gandhi. Additionally, part of this chapter uses writings by Gandhi when he was in South Africa. This was a period when he was actively involved with sanitary work, following epidemics of plague and smallpox and non-infectious diseases like malaria. In order to comment on Gandhi's notions of contagion, filth, national identity, class, and caste issues, I have used his writings from the period when he was in South Africa between 1893 and 1914. This highlights Gandhi's transnational political career, an important dimension of which involved sanitary reform work.

Body, affect, and Gandhi

Gandhi, his life and his work have been the focus of a recent spurt of interdisciplinary scholarship that has revisited some of the theoretical, methodological, and historiographical concerns that characterized earlier work on him. The journal *Public Culture* printed an issue on the one hundredth anniversary of Gandhi's seminal text *Hind Swaraj*, the central premise of which was to focus on the movability and transportability of Gandhi, his ideas and his writings across the globe. The contributors challenge the intellectual assumptions within which much of the historical scholarship on Gandhi was framed, and focus on *Hind Swaraj* to that end. *Hind Swaraj*, which according to Arjun Appadurai is a truly 'diasporic text', has had a rich afterlife, whereby it has opened itself up to a number of new contexts and interpretations.

The text and the man who wrote it, argue the contributors, should both be revisited and reevaluated. What is interesting about this new body of work is that the essays are neither staunch about 'attention to contextualization', nor about the 'biography' that 'characterizes the life of the saint'.[4] The goal was to read Gandhi's texts, especially *Hind Swaraj*, in a more flexible and open-ended way so that they can address new agendas that reflect the importance of Gandhi in our contemporary lives. As the editors say,

> The *swaraj* that Gandhi struggled to attain challenged the distinction between individual and collective and thus was available to

anyone at any time without any recourse to some historical or ideological telos.[5]

This chapter owes a great deal to some other seminal work on Gandhi as well. In an innovative move, there has been a shift away from studying Gandhi as the quintessential national leader or Mahatma, the saintly political guru of modern India. Scholars have been more interested in knowing Gandhi through other aspects of his life as well, be they his friendships or his fasts. The most noteworthy contribution is Joseph Alter's monumental *Gandhi's Body: Sex, Diet, and the Politics of Nationalism*. Bringing down Gandhi from a rarefied realm of lofty political ideals to a more grounded way of reflecting on his everyday practices is the explicit objective of this fascinating text. Alter offers a nuanced critique of Gandhi, the man, through his trials and failures in his corpus of bodily experiments. For this chapter, I locate myself within Alter's arguments where he uses the body to rethink the career of the Mahatma. As Alter argues,

> [T]he body as a whole is simultaneously a concrete aspect of material culture and an organism situated in the natural order of things. Thus, the body as a whole is, all at once, a sensory self, a product of history, and a thing of nature. What this means is that the body, and the concepts of embodiment and body discipline – unlike the concepts of identity and ideology – more clearly encode and refer to the question of 'being human' as against the question of how a human being expresses culture.[6]

And in the particular case of Gandhi, Alter finds his commitment to 'Truth' inextricably linked his bodily capabilities and limits. He quotes Gandhi's statement that 'morals are closely linked to health. A perfectly moral person can achieve perfect health', arguing that morality and health were the two sides of Gandhi's politics.

Alter is undoubtedly one of the first scholars to consider Gandhi's commitment to health worthy of intellectual analysis and make it his analytical point of departure. Instead of treating Gandhi's biomorality as derivative, Alter squarely situates health and hygiene as centerpieces of Gandhi's life and politics.[7] Taking that argument forward, my chapter argues that matters of health, hygiene, and sanitation go into the heart of Gandhi's understanding of caste, class, and nationhood. In his short essay in *The Story of My Experiments with Truth* called 'Sanitary Reform and Famine Relief', Gandhi writes:

> Ever since my settlement in Natal, I had been endeavoring to clear the community of a charge that had been levelled against it, not without a certain amount of truth. The charge had often been made that the Indian was slovenly in his habits and did not keep his house and surroundings clean.[8]

Being clean and practicing sanitary habits were central to Gandhi's idea of an enlightened community. He chronicled the deep bitterness he experienced while trying to influence public opinion within the Indian community in Natal about the need to initiate sanitary reforms. 'At some places I met with insults, at others with polite indifference. It was too much for people to bestir themselves to keep their surroundings clean'.[9] The feelings of frustration and dismay are unmistakable here. He went on to say that it was the reformer who suffered all the agony in order to initiate reforms. The community was indifferent and hostile at times and completely disregarded the anguish such responses caused the reformer. What is striking, however, is the connection he made between his appeals for such endeavors on the behalf of the Indian community and what he called his own 'self purification'. He emphasized to the diasporic Indian the value of contributing to the Motherland in the form of sanitary relief work. Sanitation was therefore central to questions of selfhood not only for Gandhi himself but for the community as well.

The table of contents in *The Story of My Experiments with Truth* is evidence of the centrality of all issues related to health and hygiene to Gandhi's broader political project, beginning in South Africa. Titles like 'The Black Plague I and II', 'More Experiments with Dietetics', 'Fasting', and 'Fasting as Penance' run through the entire book and reiterate over and over again that health and sanitation comprise the crux of Gandhi's political desires. As Alter shows,

> [N]onviolence was, for him, as much as issue of public health as one of politics, morality, and religion. To read ahimsa (nonviolence) simply as practical philosophy, political theory, ethical doctrine, or spiritual quest is to misunderstand the extent to which Gandhi embodied moral reform and advocated that reform's

embodiment in terms of public health, which was inherently political, spiritual, and moral in the context of late imperialism.[10]

Alter rightly points out that, for example, Gandhi's *Key to Health* should be appreciated not because it was the creation of a genius 'mind' but because it held the prospects of a 'great nation'. Tanika Sarkar has also commented on the 'absorbing' and 'enduring' nature of Gandhi's preoccupation with the disciplining of the body by means of food and other healing techniques. As Sarkar says,

> He advised others about diet and medicine at enormous length. Each time he refused medicine that included ingredients he felt were forbidden on religious grounds and faced death, it was a major triumph of will, an affirmation of his moral power, his claim to leadership. The regimes could never stabilize, requiring, instead, unending attention and vigilance, as he improvised fresh privations and new modes of diet and medicine. The innovations provided the core of his care of the self.[11]

It is only in tandem with his politics of the body that one can appreciate Gandhi's politics of feelings and affect as well. If *swaraj* or self-rule entailed manipulation and mastery over the body and its physiological processes, such dominance was in essence command over the fluctuations of emotions as well. In fact, for Gandhi, one's affective life held the key to one's corporeal life and emotions controlled bodily processes. As Tanika Sarkar says, 'The body, like the inner self, had to be pared down to the bones, brought, practically to its vanishing point. His approach toward a body with needs was unforgiving.'[12] The process of reducing the body to a skeletal but resilient basis was to be achieved by the manipulation of affects. If the body constituted the kernel of his politics, his politico-moral and political journey can be read as a narrative in affective transactions he entered into with the modern Indian nation, and ultimately with himself. If having supreme power over the body was one axis of Gandhian *swaraj*, the other axis was that of possessing an authority over certain affective uncertainties and prohibiting others altogether, especially greed, fear, and sexual pleasure.

Another piece of scholarship that I find immensely helpful in locating this chapter is Ajay Skaria's essay on Gandhi's ideas on life, living, and death, and the relationship between the *satyagrahi* and death. In an essay titled 'Living by Dying', Ajay Skaria explores the contradiction in Gandhi's conception of *dayabal* (the power of compassion) and *satyagraha*.¹³ For Gandhi, while *daya* could not be given up as long as one was alive, the practice of *daya* required the *satyagrahi* to be ready to surrender life. I read Skaria's formulation of compassion not only as moral ideal but affective as well, wherein the somatic/sensual becomes intertwined with the purely emotional. The following quote from one of Gandhi's texts, *The Good Life*, illustrates this precise connection between the sensual, physical, affective, and moral. Gandhi writes,

> The next is gradual control of the senses. A *Brahmachari* must control his palate. He must eat to live, and not for enjoyment. He must only see clean things and close his eyes before anything unclean... A *Brahmachari* will likewise hear nothing obscene or unclean, smell no strong, stimulating things. The smell of clean earth is far sweeter than the fragrance of artificial scents and essences. Let the aspirant to *Brahmacharya* also keep his hands and feet engaged in all the waking hours in healthful activity. Let him also fast occasionally. The third step is to have clean companions, clean friends and clean books.¹⁴

This particular has helped me to locate Gandhi's engagement with the body, and his understanding of life, death, and health. Gandhi was unique in his unwillingness to grant life as the biggest gift to human beings. Preserving life by unfair, sinful, or violent means was unacceptable to him. For him the power of the *satyagrahi* came precisely from his or her ability to give up life.

Gandhi's fasts

One of Gandhi's first pieces on fasting at the Tolstoy Farm in South Africa described it thus:

> Having been born in a Vaishnava family and of a mother who was given to keeping all sorts of hard vows, I had observed, while in India, the Ekadashi, and other fasts, but in doing so I had merely copied my mother and sought to please my parents. At that time

I did not understand, nor did I believe in, the efficacy of fasting. But seeing that the friend I have mentioned was observing it with benefit, and with the hope of supporting the *brahmacharya* vow, I followed his example and began keeping the Ekadashi fast.[15]

Gandhi's account of this fast sets the stage for the many fasts that were to follow in his career as a political-spiritual leader. In this short essay, he described how the Hindu, Muslim, Christian, and Parsi residents of the farm welcomed the fast despite different religious, and therefore different dietary, preferences. Gandhi persuaded the 'Musalman youngsters' to observe 'ramzan' fast. Gandhi wrote about his appreciation for those youngsters since many of them were new to fasting and he cherished the fact that he could convince them of the value of fasting as a means of self-restraint. In this piece, Gandhi established the relationship between fasting, 'passions' of the flesh, and self-control. Fasting was supposed to curb affections of the flesh and the only way that could be achieved was to internalize the spirit of self-discipline. He wrote,

> Fasting and similar discipline, is therefore, one of the means to the end of self-restraint, but it is not all, and if physical fasting is not accompanied by mental fasting, it is bound to end in hypocrisy and disaster.[16]

A reading of Gandhi's successive fasts illustrates the moral, spiritual, and, I would add, affective trials that constituted his moral and political career. Contentment, the pleasure of success, and the pain of failure are evident in his writings on the fasts. Regarded by him as one of the most formidable weapons of *ahimsa* (nonviolence) and *swaraj* (self-rule), Gandhi observed around 17–18 major fasts between 1918 and 1948.[17] Many of these fasts were tied to particular political demands at times of critical national events and his fasts acted as catalysts for political intervention. One of the most noteworthy was the September 1932 fast protesting the British government's move to set up a separate electorate on the basis of caste in India.

Gandhi undertook fasts as correctives not only for his own actions but those of others as well. For example, he wrote of another fast he undertook as a 'penance' for the failings of two Ashram inmates. This narrative is a chronicle of a deeply affective realm that was created in the wake of this fast. The reason behind this fast (the failure of the Ashram residents) contributed to the intensity of affect that surrounded it. And the degree to which Gandhi was affected by the moral collapse in the Ashram also augmented the emotional nature of that moment. Let me quote Gandhi at length.

> Once when I was in Johannesburg I received tidings of the moral fall of two of the inmates of the Ashram. News of an apparent failure or reverse in the *Satyagraha* struggle would not have shocked me, but this news came upon me l like a thunderbolt...So I imposed upon myself a fast for seven days and a vow to have only one meal a day for a period of four months and a half...My penance pained everybody, but it cleared the atmosphere...It may be recalled that during the whole of this period of penance I was a strict fruitarian. The latter part of the second fast went fairly hard with me. I had not then completely understood the wonderful efficacy of the *Ramanama*, and my capacity for suffering was to that extent less.[18]

The rest of the fast proved tough for Gandhi as he became very weak and could hardly speak. The excerpt above establishes the relationships between food and consumption, the body, self-control, and suffering that for Gandhi were central to moral membership of nation and society. The emotional anguish he suffered in the wake of the moral lapse of the Ashram residents, and the physical strain he experienced during the course of the second fast, were not just moral torment. They were deeply emotive too. What he labeled as failures to hold on to his vow steadfastly always exceeded what he could express in words and were therefore affective. The fast opened up the possibility of what Ben Highmore would call 'new sensual worlds' – emergences that would create the basis for new personal and political possibilities. Within the culture of food and religion in India, Gandhi's fasts acquired a new kind of significance by being the progressive steps from ruling the self to *swaraj*.

Race and Gandhi's politics of hygiene

The *Swachh Bharat Campaign* (Clean India Mission) inaugurated by the Prime Minister of India, Narendra Modi, in October 2014 has been a dazzling affair with celebrities from the fields of cinema, politics, and sports lending their glitz to this public health campaign. The logo of the campaign is an image of a pair of Gandhi's spectacles. Onto each of the lenses are inscribed the two words *swachh* (clean) and *Bharat* (India) and a caption below reads *Ek Kadam Swachhata Ki Ore* (One Step towards Cleanliness). It almost seems as though Gandhi is looking through his glasses at this new initiative and each lens is a window to defining, understanding, and executing each of its constitutive entities – *swachh* and *Bharat*. The goals of the campaign are ending the manual scavenging still widespread in India, eliminating open defecation, and creating awareness among the public about sanitation and its linkages to public health. The campaign has a vision of creating a 'Clean India' by 2019.

The *Swachha Bharat Abhiyan* seems a fitting tribute to Gandhi's involvement with and commitment to sanitation and public health as edifices of his political *swaraj*. In 1935 he wrote:

> Village tanks are promiscuously used for bathing, washing clothes and drinking and cooking purposes. Many village tanks are also used by cattle. Buffaloes are often to be seen wallowing in them. The wonder is that, in spite of this sinful misuse of village tanks, villages have not been destroyed by epidemics. It is the universal medical evidence that this neglect to ensure purity of the water supply of villages is responsible for many of the diseases suffered by the villagers.
>
> (*Harijan*, 1935)

Gandhi's pledge to highlight the centrality of sanitation to economic and social development and dedicate himself to this cause was for him an innately political goal. And he was very categorical in highlighting this goal:

> The task of rural sanitation is no easy one, it means nothing less than raising the village *Bhangi* to the status of an ideal *Bhangi*. The whole subject is unexplored; the profession, far from being a dirty one, is a purifying, life-protecting one. Only we have debased it. We have to raise it to its true status.
>
> (*Harijan*, 1936)

This section narrates the history of some of Gandhi's engagements with sanitary relief work and reflects on his notions of social and moral contagion. The narrative begins in South Africa with his relief work in cities like Durban, Johannesburg, and Natal. As Isabel Hofmeyr has traced Gandhi's 'printing and publishing experiments' to Durban and other cities in South Africa, so were his public health experiments. To my mind, the exact same kinds of reasons that enabled him to start his experiments with publishing and printing, worked for his sanitary work as well. Hofmeyr's description is apt in this regard:

> Durban was home to a jumble of diasporic communities from different parts of the world, an environment that obliged its inhabitants to experiment with who they were or could become. Part of the vast migrations of the nineteenth century, these flows of indentured laborers, migrant workers, prisoners, sailors, pilgrims, merchants, and missionaries coalesced around the Indian Ocean littoral, in port cities (and their hinterland capitals) like Cape Town, Johannesburg, Zanzibar, Mombasa, Nairobi, Port Louis, or Bombay. In these destinations, Africans, Middle Easterners, Southeast Asians, Chinese, and Indians found themselves as happenstance neighbors, relating both to a colonial authority and to each other... While these transoceanic projects evinced cosmopolitan elements, they equally constructed distinct boundaries whether of 'race', civilization, religion, or class.[19]

In an article that was published in the *Times of India*, Gandhi chronicled the goings-on in the wake of a rumor that an Indian man had contracted the bubonic plague and died in Middleburg in Transvaal.[20] Gandhi expressed his contempt for the draconian quarantine measures that the government immediately imposed on the Indian community without proper consideration. Even internal travel by Indians was strictly restricted. A number of things happened. There was an alert throughout South Africa, Indians traveling from Mauritius, Madagascar, or an infected district in India were stopped, the quarantine measures were 'stringent', 'unreasonable', 'oppressive', and 'unbusinesslike', and business interests were seriously affected. Gandhi commented on the paradox that came out into the open once that event became widely reported: while on the one hand there was a high demand for Indian indentured labor in that region, on the other hand, for the rest of the population, strict limitation of the movements of Indians was not as problematic.

He expressed indignation at the people of South Africa for not thinking about the Indian people. He found the woes of Indian storekeepers, businessmen, and other Indian residents experienced at the hands of the governments unacceptable. Toward the end of the essay Gandhi explained the reason behind such hostilities met by Indians as an anti-Indian prejudice, which was the result of 'trade jealousy' on the part of both South Africans and the British government. He brought to task not only the colonial, white, British government but South Africans as well. A piece about plague rumors when read more closely opens up Gandhi's advocacy for the Indian community in South Africa and hints at his own racialist attitudes toward the South Africans, which scholars like Antoinette Burton have explored in fascinating detail.[21]

Several articles in the *Indian Opinion*, for example, offer accounts of Gandhi's involvement in and fights with different authorities, both British colonial and South African, to demand rights for immigrant Indians in South Africa. Demands for relief during disease outbreaks, improving filthy and unsanitary conditions in Indian neighborhoods, demands for public health infrastructure and fair immigration policies, and the problem of racial injustice toward Indians by the British government and South African people became recurring issues that Gandhi addressed.

Gandhi's initially mild prejudice against South Africans became much more pronounced subsequently. By 1904, such prejudice was quite strikingly apparent in his writings on the plague epidemic and the continued harassment of Indians under British imperial policies. What is striking in this set of articles published originally in the *Indian Opinion* is Gandhi's anger at the apparent discrimination made between Indians and the 'Kaffirs', who were 'left untouched', because they were wanted by Europeans for their labor.[22] It is hard to distinguish which outraged him more – the high handedness of the British government for their stringent administrative policies toward Indians or the fact that South Africans or 'Kaffirs' were treated better than Indians. It is important to recognize the role that race played in Gandhi's politics of hygiene in South Africa and undoubtedly in Gandhi's future political endeavors as well. In an article called, 'A Lesson from the Plague', Gandhi writes,

Such regulations, harsh as they undoubtedly are, ought not to make us angry. But we should so order our conduct as to prevent a repetition of them. And with that end in view, we should set about putting our houses in order as well literally as figuratively. The meanest of us should know the value of sanitation and hygiene. Overcrowding should be stamped out from our midst. We should freely let in sunshine and air. It short, we should ingrain into our hearts the English saying that cleanliness is next to godliness. And what then?

And what then? We do not promise that we shall at once be freed from the yoke of prejudice. A name once lost is not to be easily regained. The loss of a name is like a disease, it overtakes us in no time, but it costs us much to remove. But why need we think of reward in the shape of subsidence of prejudice? Is not cleanliness its own reward?[23]

The above excerpt is a powerful articulation of the significance of sanitation and hygiene for Gandhi's political ideals, commencing in South Africa through his work with the diasporic Indian community. It would be a mistake to read his commitment to issues of sanitation and hygiene as secondary to his political work. On the contrary, hygiene was a wellspring for Gandhi's *swaraj* and *satyagraha* later on. Hygiene, cleanliness, and sanitation are to be considered keywords to understanding Gandhi's politics with regard to race, citizenship, and belonging.[24] It also points to the transnational origins of Gandhi's Indian nationalist politics.[25] Gandhi continued to report on malaria and smallpox outbreaks in Durban and Johannesburg in 1905 in the *Indian Opinion* and emphasized the maintenance of strict sanitary rules within the Indian community.[26]

Medicine as contagion

'Medical science', Gandhi wrote in 1909, 'is the concentrated essence of Black Magic. Quackery is infinitely preferable to what passes for high medical skill' (*Hind Swaraj*, 1909). It was not that Gandhi was against medical science and for magic and quackery. He did, however, have a deep distrust of medical science, particularly of medical science becoming a panacea for everything at the cost of a person's relationship with his or her body. He exhorted:

It is our habit, that, at the slightest illness, we rush at once to a doctor, *vaidya*, or *hakim*. And if we do not, we take whatever medicine the barber or our neighbor suggests. It is our belief that no sickness can be cured without drugs. This however, is sheer superstition.

(*Indian Opinion*, 1913)

In *Hind Swaraj*, which is constructed as a dialogue between a Reader and an Editor, there is a chapter called the 'The Condition of India: Doctors', which is a conversation about ills of modern medicine. Medicine was a 'parasitical' modern profession for him. He argued that his viewpoint was not merely idiosyncratic but an expression of the wisdom of many people who felt that modern medicine was the biggest poison. For Gandhi, medicine was the biggest disruption to a person's organic relationship with his or her body. Medicine interrupted the course of a disease and its natural effects on the body. It hampered the body's own ability to fight a sickness. But what troubled Gandhi most was a moral issue. Medicine, by curing an individual of his or her symptoms, enabled the person to continue committing the same kinds of 'vices' that caused the disease in the first place. He wrote, 'I have indulged in vice, I contract a disease, a doctor cures me, the odds are that I shall repeat the vice'.[27] His strong disdain for hospitals is striking as well.

For Gandhi hospitals were spaces that propagated 'sin'. His scathing criticism of European doctors was particularly evident. 'European doctors are the worst of all. For the sake of a mistaken care of the human body, they kill annually thousands of animals. They practice vivisection'.[28] Gandhi's otherwise conciliatory tone toward the British/Europeans in the vast section of his writings and certainly his early politics is replaced by a much more straightforwardly indignant one. One recalls that in the first few lines of *Hind Swaraj*, Gandhi was explicitly critical of modernity's single-minded commitment to anything that could prolong life, whatever the goal or means. Medicine to him was one of the most potent weapons that modernity had used against humanity.[29]

One can see how for Gandhi, the human body and the body politic were intimately connected. For one to thrive, the other had to exist as well. It is important to appreciate the co-existence of the two in the very conception of Gandhian politics. That is why, be it in *Hind*

Swaraj or *The Story of My Experiments with Truth*, the reader finds Gandhi's writings on village democracy followed by his reports on nature therapy or his dietary experiments. Such coexistence of the physical, the moral, and the political in his writings is not simply coincidental but deliberate and meaningful. This is also connected to his broader alimentary politics as well, whereby anything that was not minimal, basic, and natural was not to be ingested or introduced into the body. In the particular case of vaccines, for example, being injected with vaccines containing bovine serum or human serum was the same as consuming them and therefore a taboo as per the Hindu belief system.

In the *Indian Opinion*, Gandhi published a series of articles on health called 'General Knowledge about Health' during 1913. A number of articles at the beginning of this series were on the vital necessity of pure air, earth, and water for good health. For him these three were the foundations of true health. Gandhi defined them as both food and medicine, and there was no distinction in his conception between the two. Food enabled the smooth and salubrious functioning of the body so that the body needed no medicine; if it was in sickness, the body itself produced the necessary medicine to bring itself back to health. The distinction between food and medicine was therefore superfluous in Gandhi's paradigm.[30]

Gandhi's politics of contagion needs to be appreciated within the context of colonial public health in both South Africa and India, where the state introduced severe sanitary measures which curbed the personal and collective freedoms of people, especially immigrant Indians in the case of South Africa. These policies exhibited the rampant racism of imperial powers. Gandhi's alternative biomoral/bioethical conceptions around health, illness, cure, and care were attempts to liberate health and the individual and collective bodies from such governmental intervention. They reiterated that the body is the most primary unit of the body politic and began with both the individual as well as the community being committed to its maintenance. Given that the sources of disease and illness were scattered everywhere in modern civilization, Gandhi believed that rightful self-conduct was the only practice which could alone guarantee health. And moral self-regulation was the basis of social, political, and cultural living. Health was synonymous with civilization in Gandhian thought and as he emphatically put it, health was a reward in itself and not because it served any particular political or social need.

What is noteworthy about Gandhi's conception of contagion is that for him contagion emanated from the self or was created by the self. It was not an external threat, but a never-ending process of self-disciplining, which addressed the sources of contagion within the self. To that extent health and self-formation were coterminous. Pollution was vital in Gandhi's vocabulary of contagion and hygiene. In the context of caste Hindu beliefs, pollution could take place by any number of disruptions – physical and, more importantly, moral. While such interruptions could be external, he always emphasized that individuals should have the integrity to control such desires, both at the level of the body and the mind. Pollution could be a result of over-consumption of food, or the use of medicines for example. It could be an outcome of sexual desires or the lust for wealth. It could result from a vaccine or drinking unclean water. Exposure to some of the above-mentioned factors could be beyond an individual's control and therefore contagion would not have been prevented. Therefore, for Gandhi the goal was to empower the agent, who could stop reproducing such contagion – the individual him or herself.

4
Imagining the Social Body: Competing Moralities of Care and Contagion

Women's autobiographical writings – memoirs, diaries, and autobiographies – are no longer archival outliers. In the last 30 years historians and literary critics have enthusiastically embraced them as legitimate archival material. This chapter, drawing on this critical scholarship, explores the construction of an ethic of care within the autobiographical writings of three Bengali women during the first half of the twentieth century.

Care was a central concern in the medical debates of the early twentieth century. Debates on the emergence of nursing as a profession, which included contentious discussions over what constituted 'modern' nursing, translated care into a larger social and moral ethic at this time. This chapter examines Bengali women's autographical writings to highlight the entwined emergence and enforcements of care as a modern medical practice and care as a social and moral principle.

While care's role as a centerpiece of modern medicine is well acknowledged, its constituent role in the affective history of hygiene is less so. The ethic of care, as I show in this chapter, was a defensive response to the fear of contagion. Its affect was not self-enclosed but bound up with, and gendered by, anxiety about the circulatory properties of disease and its impact on the religious and secular 'space' of the household and the body. Care as an affective offshoot of contagion was produced in another significant way. In the writings that I examine, contagion represented the spread of social ills and as such symbolized the decay of social and moral fabric. Women often wrote about 'afflictions' such as lack of education among women and child marriage, which, they argued, doomed women's social standing, and led to a severe dearth of maternity provisions for women, which in turn led to the loss of lives of mothers and their newborn children. These 'afflictions' collectively signified lives of limitless suffering for Bengali women that needed care and attention.

Care, apart from immediate concerns with 'health', thus encompassed a number of intertwined objectives. It was framed as an ideology aimed at social and physical transformations. It also represented a political gesturing to justify, albeit implicitly, women's increasing presence in the public sphere. And, finally, care was a moral response, which, while critical of a patriarchal society and nation, emphasized the elevated morality that women could claim as a collectivity.

This chapter highlights how even when binary divisions such as colonizer/colonized were instituted and enforced, middle class Bengali imaginaries and practices often crossed East/West divisions, as knowledge, objects, and desires continually moved across these boundaries. Moreover, in the women's autobiographies and their writings on health, the personal and domestic and the public and national were not only entwined, but also informed each other. In particular, the chapter explores the following questions: (1) How were ideas of contagion produced and managed within the domestic sphere? (2) What role did affect play in the production and circulation of ideas of contagion? (3) How did ideas of contagion move within and outside of the domestic sphere? (4) How were memory, home, and objects brought together in the service of such projects?

The chapter is divided into four sections. The first section locates the social-political context of women's writings on care. The second section, 'Memorable objects: childhood, memory, and care in Shukhalata Rao's writings', examines affect as it framed care as a spiritual, moral, and social endeavor in early twentieth-century Bengal. Through a reading of Shukhalata Rao's memoir, *Pather Alo* ('Leading Lights'), this section traces Rao's investments in the production and circulation of care in response to social and moral contagion.

In the third section, 'Traveling memories: Wandering and care in Purnashashi Debi's autobiography', I show how an ethic of care was located also in itinerant life. Debi's social critique was deeply inflected by her forever wandering life. And her philosophy of care was inspired by events and figures that she associated with compassion and care, or their lack. The last section of this chapter, 'Memorable spaces: Suffering and the education of care in Priyabala Gupta's memoir', examines *Smritimanjusha* (A Treasury of Memories), a chronicle of her life that was motivated by a singular and powerful thirst for knowledge and an unflinching desire for education for women. Gupta's social and moral critique emerged directly out of this zeal and care, for her, as I show, was an embodied practice.

Locating women's writings on care in early twentieth-century India

Although British colonial rulers had introduced Western medical education for Indians in the 1830s, it was not until 50 years later that Indian women and their health became a focus of interest for British men and women – colonial administrators, philanthropists, and missionaries – and Indian men. The Countess of Dufferin's Fund, popularly known as the Dufferin Fund, which was established in 1885, marked the first formal attempt on the part of the Raj to extend medical assistance to Indian women. This Fund opened the *zenana*, which stood for everything that was decadent, regressive, and conservative about the gender system in India, to medical reform.[1] 'Established in 1885 by Lady Dufferin, wife of the new viceroy of India, the Dufferin Fund', as Maneesha Lal rightly asserts, 'constituted the single most important institutionalization of gender in the history of colonial medicine in India'.

This new fund was established with the explicit objectives of extending medical care to Indian women, building hospitals, and encouraging women to study medicine. It was more a philanthropic passion pursued by Christian women missionaries from Britain and the United States than a direct concern of the colonial state. The last objective was particularly daunting given the fact that medicine was stringently a male dominated profession and women who dared to study medicine had to endure stiff social pressures from their families and the community. Eventually, in 1916, an exclusively women's medical college, the Lady Hardinge Medical College, was opened in Delhi.

Meera Kosambi, through her study of the life of Anandibai Joshee, vividly illustrates the trials and tribulations of women seeking to join the medical profession. Joshee, who came from an orthodox

Brahmin family, became the first Indian doctor to qualify as a medical practitioner after she received her medical degree in the United States. The life of Kadambini Ganguly, the first female graduate and medical practitioner of Bengal, similarly highlights the immense difficulties women faced at this time. In 1886, Ganguly graduated from Bengal Medical College and was given permission to practice Western medicine in Bengal, which raised the ire of conservative Bengali Hindus, who launched a slander campaign against her.[2] Haimabati Sen's journey in pursuance of a career in medicine, as she vividly records in her memoir, was fraught with similar social hindrances.[3]

Although medicine, in the late nineteenth and early twentieth centuries, was increasingly becoming an accepted field of work for the *bhadramahila* (educated, urban, middle class women), their professional experience continued to suffer under the discriminatory policies of the colonial government.[4] English women doctors were able to take advantage of the racial discrimination of colonial rulers to monopolize all available positions, thereby considerably hampering the advancement of Indian women doctors. 'Indian women doctors', as Meredith Borthwick argues, 'were left to labor under the oppressive effects of dual discrimination on grounds of both sex and race'.[5]

During this period the demand for medical professionals was, however, increasing.[6] This demand, as Geraldine Forbes, among others, explains, was in part the result of an increasing appreciation of curative institutionalized Western medicine by middle class Indian women. Such demands also came from the manufacturing sector, which provided medical aid to its employees. Lastly, the demand for medical professionals was a result of the colonial government, which from the late nineteenth century pursued an aggressive policy of 'civilizing' the society it ruled by setting up a network of hospitals, medical schools, and dispensaries.[7] Women were thus an important element in the growth of the medical profession, though their advancement was severely restricted.

The medical profession was also marked by distinctions. While medicine became a respectable profession for educated middle class Indian women, despite the ideological and structural problems that women faced, midwifery, which was commonly misused, bore a heavy burden. The majority of women, both in rural and urban India, depended on midwives for childbirth. Midwifery was a 'hereditary occupation' and midwives usually came from lower caste and class backgrounds. Midwives were popular among women for several reasons, most notably, their familiarity, easy accessibility, affordability, and shared knowledge of cultural practices around childbirth and motherhood.

Midwifery was deemed to be in urgent need of reform, both by the colonial authorities and the nationalists, because it was seen as a symbol of the degenerate state of women in India. In view of the fact that it was considered the most shameful instance of the 'domestic troubles of women in India', midwifery became a tool for colonial and nationalist interventions.[8] The Victoria Memorial Scholarship Fund, which was established in 1901–1902 to ameliorate the situation, had the specific objectives of 'training a superior class of midwives' and 'to impart a certain amount of practical knowledge to the indigenous midwives (*dais*)'.[9] Colonial authorities and missionaries commonly attributed the lack of success of such programs to the ignorance of midwives and their resistance to modernization. They also explained the lack of success, at least partly, by the structural inadequacies of these programs, for example, lack of funds, dearth of secluded wards that could attract upper caste women, and lack of medical expertise.

The already highly charged anxiety about the 'offensive' practices of ignorant midwives was further aggravated with concerns over child health and development. As a result, the Lady Chelmsford All India League for Maternity and Child Welfare was created. The League was aimed at creating awareness about child health, training health visitors, educating women at home, and creating a body of health inspectors, who visited schools to evaluate the standards of hygiene practiced within them.[10]

Concerns about infant mortality and midwifery were not unique to the colonial context. From the late nineteenth century onwards, rising infant mortality captured the attention of the British authorities in India as well as England. In the context of India, this 'vast' problem was attributed to the *dais* – the local midwives – who were not formally educated in maternal and childcare. In the mid-1920s the Association of Medical Women in India became increasingly vocal about the need to address the problem of infant mortality, calling it the 'the most sensitive index of social welfare and of sanitary administration, especially under urban conditions'.[11]

Issues of motherhood and child health were the new apologies for the empire. It was argued that the situation regarding infant mortality was particularly dismal in Bengal. Though the working class had come under scrutiny, the situation in relation to the Bengali middle class was equally bleak. The 1921 Census, for example, showed that even among the *bhadralok* the rate of infant mortality was double the corresponding figure in Europe.[12] In the popular imperial vocabulary, therefore, motherhood and childhood became the entwined centerpieces of a debate that revolved around the future of the nation.

These concerns actively framed early twentieth-century Indian feminism as well. Women's political activism on issues such as the vote was equally committed to the cause of women's health and physical culture, for example. Significantly, Kadambini Ganguly, the first woman medical practitioner from Bengal, and Swarnakumari Devi, who is credited with founding a women's organization called Sakhi Samiti, were two of the delegates for the 1889 session of the Indian Congress in Bombay. Sakhi Samiti, an association of female friends, was designed to facilitate cooperation among women, whose lives were confined to the private sphere, by providing financial support to poor, unmarried, and widowed women.

Saraladevi Chaudhurani, Swarnakumari's daughter, another enthusiast for women's rights, founded the Bharat Stri Mahamandal, the first all India women's organization, in 1901. Chaudhurani also established Bharat Stri Sikhsha Sadan in Calcutta and introduced games with batons and swords among women, thereby seeking to encourage a strong ethic of physical culture among women. The rationale behind calls for the fully fledged induction of women into the political realm was that women were integrally linked to the future of the nation through their indispensable role as mothers.[13]

Health and family welfare activities were also a central concern for other women's organizations such as the All India Women's Conference (AIWC) and the Women's Indian Association (WIA). WIA under Annie Besant established maternity welfare activities from around the 1920s.

> This was taken up by the Baby Welcome Centres which were leading the way in the work of maternity and child welfare, the end in view being that the local authorities should ultimately take up this duty of educating parents and providing a suitable environment for the coming generation.[14]

Health and hygiene, defined within the parameters of motherhood and childcare, thus became feminist issues. They also became part of the broader modernist agenda in which 'domesticity and its practical forms came under even more intense surveillance in late colonial India, where the evidence [was] that home was critical to debates about how modernity could and should be played out' (pp. 8–9). In the following sections I chart the complex terrain of these debates through the writings of three well-known women medical practitioners, activists, and authors, who occupied distinctly different social positions, and yet each in their own way immensely contributed to issues of women's health and wellbeing.

Memorable objects: Childhood, memory, and care in Shukhalata Rao's writings

Shukhalata Rao belonged to an esteemed family in Bengal. She was the daughter of the well-known writer, painter, and technologist–entrepreneur Upendrakishore Ray Chowdhury. A prominent figure in the liberal Brahmo movement, Upendrakishore was revered for his pioneering work in the field of photographic reproduction, most notably the half tone print. Shukhalata Rao was the eldest daughter of Upendrakishore and a prominent literary figure herself. Educated in Calcutta, she later moved to Cuttack, Orissa with her husband Jayanta Rao.

Shukhalata Rao was involved in a variety of social work projects, for example, Sishu-O-Matri Mangal Kendra (Centre for the Welfare of Children and Mothers) and Orissa Nari Seva Sangha (Orissa Women's Welfare Centre). Rao's memoir, which I examine in the following, is unique because of its composition in verse. Titled *Pather Alo* (Leading Lights), this chronicle was penned by Rao sometime after 1937.[15] It is a set of recollections from her life, including about events from her childhood, people with whom she felt an intimacy, and times that left a deep imprint on her.

Arranged in small and medium length verses the lyrical form of this memoir is striking. The verses are presented thematically and the theme often bestows form to those verses. Hence, for example, in a segment titled 'Chalachchitra' (Cinema), the verses are presented as if a kaleidoscope of images was moving in front of someone's eyes from one end to the other. Each 'image' (verse) captures the memory of something or someone that inhabited Rao's past – for instance, her grandmother's passion for home decoration with souvenirs and curios purchased in England, and the home of her childhood, which was assured by her mother's presence and made unique by an assortment of tin and jars on shelves filled with cocoa, tea, sugar, or raisins. Another set of verses titled 'Paribarik' (Family) portrayed memories of colorful family members and delightful happenings in her childhood. She wrote about her grandfather (*dadamoshai*), her paternal grandmother (*thakurma*), and her little brother Sukumar.

Another striking feature of Rao's memoir is the lack of linear and fixed temporality. *Pather Alo* is a canvas of Rao's life dotted with individuals and events that had a special meaning for her. *Alo*, meaning light, can also be read as that beacon which leads the reader to a path of luminous self realization, and such a divine/metaphysical quest is evident in many of her other writings as well. The book is, however, distinctly different from devotional autobiographies such as Rashsundari Debi's *Amar Jiban*.[16] The spiritualism in *Pather Alo*, and Rao's other writings, exemplified a belief in the presence of an all-powerful entity, who for Rao was the supreme being and creator of this world, who provided solace during hard times, and was omnipresent. For example, in the preface to *Pather Alo*, she writes,

> I say unusual, not supernatural. Every happening always follows the law of nature. Each human soul is preserved within the supreme Almighty. Within this arrangement, each soul is connected to the other. In the same way one hears different sound waves in different environments, one soul can sense another's thought streams. This is a tested truth. When in need, the unprepared soul can always be readied. Who does that, who knows?

Rao then narrates how one day while cleaning her bedroom she heard a pigeon fluttering its wings in the adjacent room. The domestic helper brought the pigeon to her. She felt that there was a purpose behind that occurrence, since a pigeon was always a messenger. She wondered: What news was the pigeon carrying? She felt a jolt inside and right then she witnessed a soft light in the sky. In that light she saw an image of someone lying on a sick bed, their face hidden, but the border of the latter's saree visible in the fold. The person lying on the sick bed raised her hand and the bangles sparkled and seemed to beckon Rao eagerly. In an instant thereafter the image disappeared and the light faded. Rao realized immediately that her precious daughter was ill. Though she rushed to her ailing child, her daughter passed away moments before Rao arrived.

Rao's spiritualism saturated the details of her everyday life – in the nooks and crannies of her childhood home, in the moving shadows created at night as her father paced up and down with her little brother in his arms rocking him to sleep, and in the destiny of her daughter's death. For Rao the power of the almighty determined great sweeps of history too. *Pather Alo* is filled with descriptions of such moments and with the wonders of new times and new experiences. She recalls her amazement at science's new discoveries – electricity, the gramophone, electric lighting, trams, and the telephone, and her thrill upon riding in a motorcar for the first time. In Rao's memoir these instances of wonderment became moments to commemorate the personal and national, the material and metaphysical, and the private and the public.

Stylistically, *Pather Alo* is distinctly different when compared to other nineteenth- and early twentieth-century Bengali autobiographies and memoirs. Composed in both short and long verses, the book rejects any kind of obvious order or chronology. It makes no effort at capturing any kind of progression – be it in terms of the journey from childhood to adulthood, milestones of achievement, or evolution of a subject. Rao's memoir is much more of a wandering narrative, at least in terms of its organization. If there is one flavor that is characteristic of the book, it is this – it is an exposition of, and in, wonderment. Rao's expertise as an acclaimed children's storywriter is clearly reflected in the tone and literary techniques used in her memoir. She presents her life as the story of a journey that is filled with the wonders of her encounters with and experiences of this world and its changing landscapes. Every experience in Rao's world was filled with wonder, even when it was deeply painful.

Pather Alo is unique in another way. The reader hardly ever finds explicit articulations or traces of the anxiety and frustration that many women writers of the time expressed in their autobiographical writings. Nineteenth- and early twentieth-century women's autobiographies, especially in the context of India, in contrast to Rao's memoir, are full of tales of deprivation, suffering, and helplessness. These reflected the experiences of many women as they questioned the impositions of a patriarchal system within which they were embedded but were also revolting against, even if silently. Some of them finally broke social and cultural barriers either with the help and support of family members or completely on their own. The desire to read and write, for example, became one of the most powerful expressions of the intense struggle many women waged. It would not be an understatement to say that the desire to be literate became the paramount mission for many nineteenth-century middle class women. Rashsundari's *jitakshara* is the finest example of such a mission. Tanika Sarkar writes,

> Only one event of an exceptional kind had interrupted the even, quiet rhythms of a conventional domestic existence... In Rashsundari's own family, feelings ran so high against women's education that she would not so much as glance at a piece of paper lest she be accused of knowing how to read... This one act of disobedience, then, partially deconstructs the good wife – a script that Rashsundari otherwise followed with admirable success all her life. Why did she, on her own, and in great trepidation, make this deeply transgressive departure?[17]

The two women writers whose work I analyze later in this chapter, namely Purnashashi Debi and Priyabala Gupta, penned some of their own desires and subsequent endeavors to achieve those goals. And such concerns are strikingly absent in *Pather Alo*. The obvious reason is of course Rao's class background. She belonged to one of the most illustrious and well off families of nineteenth-century Bengal. Her father was a cultural icon and her brother Sukumar Ray was a gifted writer, poet, and playwright. Rao's husband belonged to a financially and socially established family as well. Her father-in-law Madhusudan Rao was an eminent Oriya poet and her husband Jayanta Rao was a physician by profession. For Rao, access to education, therefore, was hardly a concern. Being a part of the social and cultural elite gave Rao easy access not only to education but also to a vibrant intellectual circle, which undoubtedly influenced her own literary career.

Rao, nevertheless, shared many other concerns of women of the time. One particular trope or theme that has been persistent in many women's autobiographies and memoirs of nineteenth and early twentieth-century India has been death, and it is evident in Rao's writings as well. The emotional ordeal following the death of close family members – siblings, parents, or children – often acted as a quandary, crisis, and/or predicament that formed the backdrop for many women writers from this period. If education became a catalyst that framed the subjectivity or agency of women writers of the time, death, bereavement, and loss signified another terrain on which many women writers reflected 'new knowledge' about themselves.[18] Shukhalata Rao, for example, wrote, in the preface to *Pather Alo*:

> The compassionate almighty lord had blessed us with six children. He had taken three of them back to him. Of my three daughters, I am going to write about Manika in this short essay...She was married on 6th of May. Exactly one year after her wedding, she left this world on the same day.[19]

A similar trope is presented in Priyabala Gupta's son Ranjan Gupta's comments on his mother's memoir,

> [When] the day for Baradadu's *shraddha* (funeral rites) was still sometime away, a second death visited the family. My three-year-old elder brother died after suffering from a terrible attack of blood dysentery...There were no tube wells in our village. We all used to drink water from the village pond. People frequently suffered from intestinal illnesses...People said different things to console her. My mother hardly had any outward show of her grief. The only time she could lighten the burden of her sorrow was at night when after a long day of housework she sat down with her journal, in which she used to write her poetry – her small refuge.[20]

But perhaps nobody endured more agony from the untimely deaths of intimate family members than Purnashashi Debi. She narrated the death of her husband, which took place within six months of her brother's death. And her sister-in-law survived for only one year after her husband's death. Her heartbreaking narratives of the sudden deaths of her husband and her sister-in-law, on the one hand, reflect how family continued to be central to the life worlds of these women and yet, on the other hand, in the very articulation of these narratives these women also exemplified their independence.

The death of her husband triggered a period in Debi's life that she called 'a betrayed life' – a time of endless suffering and anguish. She writes, 'When I think of those days my heart still shudders. Many women face widowhood, but I wonder whether anyone else has had to suffer the pain, anguish, disrespect, and torment that I had to go through'.[21] Purnashashi Debi also lost three of her sons in 1950, 1961, and 1964. Arunkumar Bandyopadhyay, her grandson, writes, 'Finally when Bharat committed suicide on 16 January 1964 in a hotel at Dehri-On-Sone in Bihar, Purnashashi could not take the shock anymore. She took to bed. She even lost her faith and confidence in herself'.[22]

Writings on the deaths of close family members and the attendant pain and loss cannot be abstracted from the emotional, spiritual, and moral conundrums in these women writers' engagement with and investments in producing and practicing an ethic of care. The expressions of 'extreme suffering' also provided social and moral critiques, which, however, were rarely presented explicitly as such.[23] While these writers did not commonly express the connections between their loss and a social and moral critique of a deeply patriarchal and unequal society, to overlook those linkages would be missing a crucial element of their politics. For example, Priyabala Gupta's three-year-old son's death was the result of an infection from drinking unclean water from the village pond. Her weaving in of the social context of the loss was not incidental. Gupta's commitment to poetry was paralleled by her dedication to causes of women's education and safe motherhood. This is one of many examples of how the personal became tied to a literary, social, and moral reform agenda.

To come back to my discussion of Shukhalata Rao's childhood memories, her personal tragedies, her religious predilections, and her writing practices have to be seen as meaningfully interlinked narratives. *Pather Alo* is an eloquent and lively chronicle of spaces, times, events, and objects that crowded Sukhalata's past. Rao moves deftly between different kinds of spaces and events in her narratives and, as I mentioned earlier, there is no fixed and linear temporality to the descriptions either. For example, she recounted the time when her maternal grandmother, Kadambini Ganguly, the first woman physician in India and one of the first Indians to graduate from Britain, returned from England: 'I remember how adorned her home was. She decorated it with beautiful dolls she brought from England'.[24]

Colonial adornments and identity were woven together with the spaces and objects that constituted the home. In one of her verses she wrote,

> the film is torn at many places, many gaps. Images surface here and there – at the market, red and blue balloons, small pots and pans to play with, buying those dolls which would nod once you turned the key; taking a bath in the water filled storage tank; and sitting in the long veranda, my mother feeding all of us from the same plate.[25]

What is striking in *Pather Alo* is the complex amalgam of objects, people, and affects that constituted Rao's field of memories. It presents, to borrow a term from Lynda Dyson, a 'mnemonic landscape' – a social and moral topography that brings objects, spaces, and affects together to create meaning and value.[26] In a very different context, elaborating the relationship between objects, values, and specific historical conjunctures, Lynda Dyson writes: 'Given that everyday habits and rituals are anchored in, and crystallized around, the use and display of artefacts, the day to day processes of social reproduction endow objects with new and different meanings'.[27] 'The spatialized landscape of everyday objects', Dyson elaborates, 'plays a central role in organizing the textuality of memory from which autobiographical narratives are constructed'.[28]

The amalgams of things/objects and times/events in *Pather Alo* are, similarly, reflective of how identities like gender, class, caste, religion, and nation are produced at the interstices of the everyday lives of individuals and the nation(s). The list of objects/things that give life to Rao's past is a testimony of her entrenchment in an upper middle class Brahmo family and her investments in the cultural production of a modern Indian home, family, and nation. In her memories we see 'how everyday objects became part of her inner life' and simultaneously reflective of an imagination for a modern and progressive cultural and social collective life.[29]

Rao's cultural and social politics and her understanding of contagion and the ethic of care crucially informed each other. And this becomes evident when Rao's memoir *Pather Alo* and a collection of writings titled *Swasthya* (Health) are read together. *Swasthya*, which was published in 1922, was recommended reading for children in primary school. It is an illustrated commentary on the basic tenets of hygiene and wellbeing. It emphasizes the importance of early rising, the value of taking a bath every day, the meanings of hygiene, food, and nutrition, the necessity of physical exercise, and the cleanliness of one's home and surroundings.

Swasthya is presented as a conversation between a mother, a father, and their four children, Malati, Sunil, Sudhir, and P(n)utu. Marked by the use of simple and accessible language, this didactic text was primarily instructive in nature. Through these lessons, Rao defines hygiene and health as a set of practical habits and seeks to induct children as agents for the foreseen transformation. For the first edition of *Swasthya*, Dr Chunilal Basu, a Bengali physician known for his writings on personal hygiene and health, especially the role of food in health and wellbeing, wrote the preface. Basu played an important role in debates on food and nutrition and food policies in colonial Bengal. What is noteworthy in Basu's preface is the words of praise he has for a booklet on health and hygiene written for school children. He had been persistently voicing concerns over the dwindling health of Bengalis, their very limited or absent knowledge of modern hygiene, and the widespread existence of contagious diseases. Basu's praise for this booklet, written for school children in the lucid vernacular, emphasized the wider intersections of such concerns at this time.

Swasthya, apart from its focus on children, was a typical early twentieth-century pedagogic text on personal hygiene, similar types of which had flooded the Bengali print market. It deploys distinctly modern nineteenth-century public health language in which water, air, filth, and odor were central to any discourse on contagion. Notions of germs and miasma were incorporated within a paradigm that focused on public health as a combination of science, skills, and beliefs.[30] In the text, the four siblings and their friends, in the course of their daily lives around school and play, end up with small illnesses, injuries, and indispositions. Solutions and remedies are provided as these four siblings and their parents offer and explain them in the language of modern hygiene and medicine.

Swasthya was an expression of Rao's bourgeois, modern, Bengali middle class sensibilities that linked hygiene and health organically to liberal notions of familial life. The theme that runs through *Swasthya* is contagion and its relation to habit, order, and practice. The anecdotes compiled in this text outline how contagion happens, the outcomes of contagion, and how to counteract it. The text, emphasizing the process of contagion, frames contagion through a series of oppositions – *jibanu* (germ)/*beej* (seed) and hygiene/cleanliness/disinfection. In these oppositions one set of notions, for example germs/negativity/adversary, is posited against the other, hygiene/positivity/ally.

In one of the anecdotes, Sudhir wakes up with a swollen face and severe toothache and his father explains what causes toothache and how the germ/seed destroys teeth, and in the process the basic features of dental hygiene are presented. In another anecdote, Malati's friend Usha comes to see her, but Usha's sister, Sushila, who also wanted to visit Malati, is not able to do so because of high fever from malaria. Malati's mother explains why the small water reservoir beside their house could be a breeding ground for mosquitoes that carry the malaria germ/seed and thereafter she goes on to elucidate what could be done about it.

In these narratives Bengali concepts and practices get suffused with Western/scientific/English terms. Contagion, for example, is explained through contact and the contiguity of physical spaces and material objects, but is also recast in moral and affective terms. Contagion could be a menace; it could, however, be checked by the inculcation of correct social and moral values and habits that were also modern. Health hazards could thus be countered with another 'contagion' – that of modern hygiene – thereby remaking contagion as an outbreak of modern social and cultural values and practices. Rao's ethic of care brought together knowledge, body, and habit.

Care, for Rao, was a thoroughly embodied process that needed to acquire and incorporate new knowledges and transform them into the habits of everyday life. Care was, however, a social habit that was simultaneously physical as well as moral and cultural. Such holistic folding together of bodily and spiritual, knowledge and values, and habits and learning into an ethic of care can be discerned if we read Rao's autobiography together with her writings on health. Putting together *Swasthya* and *Pather Alo* also enables us to appreciate Rao's principle of care as a crucial element of her early twentieth-century social feminist ideology and practice.

Memorable spaces: Suffering and education of care in Priyabala Gupta's memoir

Smritimanjusha (The Treasure House of Memories), a compilation of Priyabala Gupta's writings, is one of a large number of stories, memoirs, and autobiographies in Bengali by nineteenth- and twentieth-century women writers that have been recently compiled, edited, and republished by the Women's Studies Department of Jadavpur University, Calcutta, India. These compilations are an archival treasure trove of women's writings that explore the meanings and value this time had for these women, the challenges they faced, and the spirit with which they attempted to overcome some of those challenges.

The republished volumes, along with a selection of author's writings, usually have a biography of the author and an introduction by people who have closely followed these authors' work, sometimes a relative of theirs. While some of these female authors became well known as writers, novelists, or social reformers, many remained relatively unknown. Often these women pursued writing careers while waging struggles against hierarchical social institutions and other forms of subjection.

One of the goals of this retrieval project has been to introduce lesser-known female literary figures and locate them and their work within the cultural and social histories of colonial and postcolonial Bengal. According to the founding director of the School of Women's Studies, Jadavpur University, Jasodhara Bagchi, 'these autobiographies are a testimony of the imprint of a gendered social structure on the lives and psyche of these women. They are not only an expression of [their] deprivation, but their capabilities as well'.[31]

Bagchi, in the preface of *Smritimanjusha*, states: 'Priyabala Gupta never became famous'. However, she 'was revered within her family and her village for her knowledge and humanitarianism'. Although Gupta suffered from anxieties as a result of her father's traveling career during her childhood, this was also a happy time, because Gupta could pursue her studies. 'The school signified an expanding world of knowledge despite the thousand barriers' she faced. However, her family's concern with her marriage, when she was just 13 years old, dramatically changed her life. 'For Priyabala, the biggest tragedy of her life was when her education was discontinued, in consideration of her marriage prospects'.[32]

'I used to dream', Priyabala Gupta writes in her autobiography, 'that after my marriage I would enter a world full of bliss and would be able to pursue my studies'.[33] But, she says,

> I could not find their slightest trace in reality. So much of desire had I harbored. I could not tell anyone here what a great blow it was to my dreams. Who would even understand? Trying to explain [to] someone would have brought a bigger trouble. Moreover I was too young to explain to others or follow a path of my choosing.[34]

Gupta 'harbored a deep hurt all her life against her father, who once had encouraged her to study and develop her poetic abilities. But changed completely once she was of marriageable age'.[35] Gupta's life experiences, in a significant way, were in stark contrast to those of Shukhalata Rao, though both had to confront gendered and patriarchal practices. Nevertheless, Gupta did not give up. Her experiences left a deep imprint on her and she realized that 'the fundamental cause behind all ills, especially those, which constrained women, was upper caste and upper class Hindu conservatism'. She did not abandon reading and writing. 'Her poetic accomplishments, promotion of education for women, [and] commitment to helping and educating women in the correct lessons of maternal care within the material and ideological constraints of everyday life made her exceptional'. Lack of literacy, poor sanitary conditions, and 'the horror of aturghar' (a traditional birthing room) in her village troubled her. She learnt midwifery and used her skills to positively transform the infant mortality situation in her village.[36]

Interestingly, while transitioning into married life caused the biggest disruption in Gupta's life, because she had to leave her studies, she perceptively, and also poignantly, interwove her own experiences with the tumultuous political climate of the time, particularly with the *swadeshi* movement:

> I soon arrived at my marriageable age, and my studies came to a stop. This was also the time of Swadeshi. The revolutionary time had sounded its war bugle and the skies and air of Bengal breathed fire. Names like Khudiram, Ullashkar, Prafulla Chaki were chanted even by the children of Bengal. There was tremendous excitement in the hearts of the people of Bengal. Everywhere there

were meetings and arrests, deaths by hanging, bonfires of foreign textiles, 30 Ashwin – the day of token stoppage of all domestic cooking, Rakshabandhan, and singing Swadeshi songs. Caught in the midst of all this ferment, my studies were swept away like a small twig in a frothing stream.[37]

The abrupt interruption in Gupta's studies and the historical conjuncture at which it happened became the context for *Smritimanjusha*. In the autobiography, she strongly critiques the conservative Hindu *zamindar* (landlord) family she was married into and through her life experiences also provides a critique of patriarchal customs among upper caste Hindu. What she found most distressing was that despite being *zamindars*, the village of her father-in-law was deeply backward. She writes: 'After marriage, I went to my father-in-law's house. That most residents of this village were uneducated was the first thing I noticed. No one cared about education and [they were] burdened by superstitions'.[38] Her disdain for many of the customs followed by her new family is starkly evident. She felt out of place moving in an environment where women still did not wear a chemise regularly, and she was ridiculed frequently for wearing one. This particular concern, however, was a part of the broader disappointment that she felt in living in a world without education – a world in which she, and many others like her, was not even allowed to pursue education:

> Neighbor wives and girls would come for a chat...They would leave soon with a polite goodbye...I would invite them to come again but there was no genuine eagerness. My true companions in these times were the few books I owned – *Kabya Kusumanjali*, *Kanakanjali*, and *Aryanari*, volumes one and two. My eyes would often fill up with tears when I realized that I was surrounded by abysmal darkness. Where was light? There were plenty of books here, but I lacked the courage to ask. What if they were offended? The only thing that occupied me was how to take out time so that I could read.[39]

If one had to highlight the affective, emotional, and moral centerpiece of Gupta's life, it undoubtedly would be a combination of her anguish, distress, and sadness, her pleasure in education and her single-minded passion for being able to read and write.

Smritimanjusha is remarkable in the absence of details of Gupta's domestic life. Tanika Sarkar has remarked how Rashsundari Debi's *Amar Jiban* lacks the 'concrete and the sensuous dimensions of everyday life... There are few descriptions of exterior landscapes, of domestic interiors. There is no impression of taste, sound or smell'.[40] As far as *Smritimanjusha* is concerned Priyabala Gupta similarly avoided any detailed narrative of her household life, especially after her marriage. And whenever she did engage with everyday living, it was mostly to offer a critical commentary on patriarchal customs and practices and the abject situation of women.

Domesticity is thus an absent presence in Gupta's autobiography. Nevertheless, it also forms the context, backdrop, and evidence of what Priyabala found terribly oppressive in caste Hindu families – a reality that constricted women within narrow confines, devoid of any freedom to pursue their own desires. Her own domestic life thus became a conjunction of people, ideologies, values, and everyday practices against which she evaluated the burdens of womanhood.

The two causes in which Priyabala Gupta had immersed herself were women's education and maternal health. These endeavors began when some young women from the village came to her for help in composing personal letters. 'I used to feel bad. Why don't you learn to read and write? You can then express your own thoughts yourself', she writes. But when these women asked her, 'Who would teach us to read and write?', it gave her the reason to finally give shape to her commitment to women's education, which she considered foundational for women's rights.[41] Of course 'rights' was not a term she herself used; she described them as the desires which women harbored in their hearts, but seldom had opportunities to fulfill.

In *Smritimanjusha*, Gupta also expressed horror at the state of women's health. Her own experiences with motherhood and the ordeal that many young women in the village went through during childbirth contributed directly to the disapproval she had for childbirth practices. She also deplored the general condition of health care that was available in the village. Her six-month-old son, for example, became severely sick with blood dysentery. She narrated how the little child had severe pain and the *kabiraj* was of no help. Her husband's family never availed of any other therapy apart from Ayurveda.

Gupta, instead, wanted to take her son to Dhaka (where her parents lived) for treatment by a renowned allopathic/*daktari* physician and it required a lot of convincing before she was allowed to do so. Gupta's disdain for *kabiraji* and Ayurveda is very explicit. She was similarly horrified by and critical of the existing childbirth practices:

> For a long time I harbored a deeply critical stance toward care for the mother and the new child. Village *aturghar*! What a nightmarish place that used to be. To this day I search for an appropriate word to describe its inhumanity. When I think of those terrible days of my life, I wonder how I survived those ordeals. The suffering that I endured at the hands of untrained midwives, from the time of my pregnancy till my child was delivered would forever be etched in my memory.
>
> The birthing space was usually set up right beside a fire pit. Be it summer or winter, it used to be the same arrangement. I was not allowed even a drop of water even if my throat was parched in the intense summer time lest the umbilical cord got infected. In case desperate mothers drank water out of thirst, no water container was left in the birthing room. The new mother had to stay in that room for three weeks to a month.[42]

Priyabala Gupta's critique of what she deemed archaic and brutal birthing practices and care of the newborn was, as is evident here, blunt. Her understanding of care – as a moral and social practice – needs to located within this context. Not unlike the start of her engagement with women's education, her tryst with midwifery started when she had to attend to a child's delivery alone. From then on she trained herself as a midwife and used to regularly attend complicated deliveries that could have jeopardized the lives of many women.

These engagements with women's education and health were not easy in themselves and the upper caste and upper class background of her affine family and its strict patriarchal values made it even harder for her to carry on such activities. Nevertheless, Gupta became a fierce critic of existing values and practices. She was, for example, very critical of traditional 'dais' (maids), who had no knowledge of modern hygiene. For her, these practices represented a stagnant system that had existed since time immemorial and therefore was resistant to transformation.

A large section of her memoir thus dwelt on her experiences with the childbirths she assisted with. Although she was critical of traditional practices, when it came to choosing between different therapeutic systems, she did not favor *daktari* (allopathic) medicine. Instead, she practiced homeopathic medicine and administered it free of cost to villagers, mostly women. Wherever she went she carried a standard text on homeopathy and a box of medicines. It needs emphasizing that Gupta was neither a qualified medical professional, nor a licensed midwife, nonetheless, she labored all her married life providing care and trying to stop the loss of lives due to dangerous midwifery practices.

It is also important to note a paradox at the heart of Priyabala Gupta's ethic of care. On the one hand, experiences of the pain and suffering of women, particularly during childbirth, connected her with other women in the village, however, on the other hand, her condemnation for *kabiraji*/Ayurvedic medicine reflected a class specific and modern sensibility that judged all Ayurvedic medicine and its practitioners to be regressive and outdated.

Priyabala Gupta searched for a meaningful life as she confronted everyday domesticity, consisting of obsolete customs and a living that was bereft of what she considered the greatest pleasure, namely education and learning. In this sense *Smritimanjusha* was very much an endeavor that had the pursuit of self-authentication and self-fulfillment at its core.[43] She measured her life and desires in relation to a community of women with whom she felt kinship of suffering, but she also knew that she would remain an outsider within this group until she could bring these women into the fold of her life's calling. Here the search for a purposeful life and writing about it merged with each other. And *Smritimanjusha* became the embodiment of that pursuit.

In *Smritimanjusha*, Gupta narrated spaces as contagion. Her reminiscences are full of meditation on spaces and places, most of which are described as dark, unsanitary, constricted and suffocating. The domestic as well as the village signified spaces that were in need of transformation because they stifled the desires of women and did not offer healthy possibilities. The affects that characterized her narratives of home in particular are very different from Sukhalata

Rao's memories of her own home, which as I showed earlier, were filled with wonderment and nostalgia. *Smritimanjusha* is mostly about Priyabala Gupta's life after marriage – her new social realities, her miseries and frustrations, and finally her struggles and successes with regard to women's health and education. She was often full of despair in her experiences of living and writing about those spaces.[44] Against this gloomy and dissenting portrayal of house and home one has to appreciate Priyabala Gupta's, to appropriate a phrase that Antoinette Burton uses more broadly, 'quest story'.[45]

Traveling memories: Wandering and care in Purnashashi Debi's autobiography

Purnashashi Debi's autobiography is a tale of travels and death. Titled *Mone Pare* (I Remember), it was written when she stayed in Benaras/Kashi and then in Brindaban, following her husband Pyarimohan's death in 1932. At a time when a professional literary career was unheard of, Debi was one of a handful of women writers for whom writing also became a source of livelihood. This was particularly helpful for her during her widowhood, which was also a time of economic distress.

Mone Pare consists of three sections – prabhate (morning), madhyannye (afternoon), and sayannnye (evening), which, roughly, encapsulate a chronological narrative of her life, from adolescence, to married and family life, and finally to life as a widow in Benaras and Brindaban. Debi's trials, tribulations, and achievements as a writer are tied to these accounts of her life. *Mone Pare* is unusual in its compelling deployment of travel and death – which characterized and deeply influenced Debi's emotional and literary life – as enduring and ceaseless tropes. *Mone Pare* is about travel, wandering, and the passage of life and death. It is also a travel narrative that seems to oscillate between the two above-mentioned constants of Debi's life and literary endeavors. Locating the significance of her writing career would be impossible without taking into account the innumerable journeys she took with her father and her husband and the spate of deaths of very close family members that she experienced, including those of her four children.

In her introduction to Purnashashi Debi's life and writings, Chitra Deb states that for many women literary figures, life outside Bengal enabled them to pursue their own desires more uninhibitedly. Being outside Bengal, Deb argues, freed these women from the rigid burdens of a Bengali patriarchal society and many novelists like Anurupa Debi, Ashapurna Debi, and Saratkumari Debi had flourishing literary lives outside Bengal.[46]

Purnashashi Debi states at the outset in her autobiography: 'I have forever been a wanderer'. *Mone Pare* reads like a travelogue and it is an account of her winding life-road, taking sudden turns and opening up new realities. Her journey, which began in Karnal, Punjab, as one of four children, came to an end when she died at the age of 76. She traveled sometimes with her father, sometimes with her husband, and in her later life, after the death of her husband, by herself. What is strikingly evident in *Mone Pare* is her sheer love for travel; being able to see new geographies, places, and people.

Her love for letters and writing acquired different meanings and significance as she saw new places in India for the first time or revisited a particular place after a long hiatus. *Mone Pare* is full of poetic descriptions of the places she traveled to and also, at times, settled in for certain periods of her life. Each of the narrated episodes features rich description of the set of characters and events involved, the meanings she drew from them and the place, and the way in which all these impacted on her literary creations. Debi's autobiography does not follow a strict chronological order, but, unlike Shukhalata Rao's memoir, there is a definite movement of time – from her birth to her last years – that is evident. *Mone Pare* thus begins with her childhood years in Kohat in the Northwestern Provinces of colonial India. She writes,

> When I think of it, everything which took place in my life began in Jhelum – childhood, writing, and my married life. Naturally, I remember that place – hidden far away in Punjab, relatively unknown and small, [it] is forever rooted in my memories – happy and wistful at the same time. I cannot even express the intimacy I feel with everything there – roads, houses, the marketplace, trees, rushing mountain stream, the hazy blue mountain ranges, and even the small pebbles in the stream. I remember how we used to play – my sister Saratsashi and me – searching for the philosopher's stone in the heap of riverine pebbles.[47]

Interrupting the portrayal of a happy childhood, amidst the beauty of the dry mountainous landscape, is Debi's longing to be able to learn to read and write. But that was unthinkable for a girl in those days. She details her appetite for knowledge when her elder brother goes to the British school and she craves to go and sit in the classroom like her brother.[48]

Her literary career, when it eventually took off, was deeply affected by her migratory life. On the pages of *Mone Pare* she often marveled at the 'riches' she was able to accumulate as she traveled to remote parts of the country. Yet there is also a sense of loss that comes to the surface from time to time in an otherwise celebratory account of travel and movement. She often, for example, repented being so far away from Bengal, where, she felt, she truly belonged. She often commented that in most of the places she stayed with her family, both before and after marriage, there were hardly any Bengalis. She also expresses her gratitude to her parents for inculcating a love of the Bengali language in her and her siblings and for teaching them the language so that even though they stayed away from Bengal, they were proficient in Bengali. Such an understanding of the Bengali self was often accompanied by othering of communities with whom she lived in the distant places. While describing her times in Kohat, for example, she remarks on the uncivilized and rough nature of the Pathans. She writes,

> Despite being under British rule, Pathans still dominated the Northwestern Provinces. They were acutely antagonistic toward white men and as a result this area lacked any law and order. Robberies and plunder were order of the day. Even the ordinary soldier would disobey the English officer's orders regularly. Because of his work orders, my father had to stay in that remote and dangerous place.[49]

On another occasion she writes: 'Wielding a knife came easily to Pathans. Everyone carried a knife – poor, rich, women and men'.[50] But she also adds that despite being barbaric, the Pathans were also a brave, fearless, hospitable, and fiercely loyal people. The contrast between genteel Bengali people and the fierce Pathans in Debi's narratives is striking and such othering and its ambivalent folding with the colonial projects are also evident in relation to other communities she came in contact with as she moved from place to place. Her patronizing depiction of Punjabis is telling:

> Civilization had still not arrived among the Punjabis. Therefore, despite the fact that the Creator had blessed them with beautiful looks, health, and vigor, they did not have any knowledge of how to use them appropriately.

Her mother never employed Punjabi servants because she considered the Punjabi language incomprehensible and because she thought that Punjabis had dirty habits. Debi's mother had Punjabi friends and she often expressed her wonder at the radiant beauty of Punjabi women, although, according to her, this was completely marred by the way they dressed and tied their hair. Debi's mother strongly objected to her children speaking in Punjabi and worried that her children would lose all civility in such a wild environment.[51] Her mother's values definitely left an imprint on Debi as well.

Yet it is her ambition for learning that is unmistakably central in Debi's narrative of traveling. It is the ultimate journey that seems to drive her. And unlike Piyabala Gupta, she was very lucky with regard to family support for her education. Purnashashi Debi's father appointed a teacher who gave lessons to the sisters at their home. Debi describes the excitement and wonder of those days, when she read new books. And this excitement about the exploration of new worlds has a lot of similarities with the emotions she uses to narrate her travels to new and unfamiliar places. She started reading whatever she could lay her hands on – novels, poetries, and short stories. And she took to writing with great enthusiasm and grit. Writing poetry in particular caused a lot of anxiety in her, because she felt it signified a lack, which she worked hard to overcome. She writes, 'I feel shy singing praises for myself. But I possessed endless patience and perseverance. Despite my repeated failure to write what I considered a decent piece of poetry, I labored at it. Soon I became more competent in writing poetry'.[52]

Her enthusiasm and perseverance, however, soon confronted an important barrier. Her studies were disrupted when she was married at the age of 13. She had to move to Farrukhabad, Uttar Pradesh, where she began a new life as a young bride that was consumed by the demands of domesticity. But unlike Priyabala Gupta's post-marriage experiences, Purnashashi Debi found a supportive husband in Pyarimohan. Pyarimohan encouraged Debi to pursue her interest in reading and writing. In the gendered and patriarchal society of the time such support was rare and extremely valuable for women, and Debi acknowledged it by showering praise on her husband.

Women writers often expressed deep gratitude for the support and acknowledgment they received from the men in their lives, especially their husbands. Purnashashi Debi, for example, was very moved when Pyarimohan showed a piece of her writing to a friend who exuberantly praised her poetic abilities. The response of women writers to such acknowledgments, apart from expressing gratitude, ironically also reflects their enclosure within a gendered and patriarchal social world. Debi writes, 'I was struck by his extraordinary magnanimity and I was filled with happiness, affection, and respect. I dreamt of the impossible. Would I ever become such a powerful writer?'[53] Pyarimohan thus became indispensable in the realization of Purnashashi Debi's desires, which without his support could have become distant dreams.

Reading and writing were taboos for married women and only a few, who were lucky enough to have supportive families, were ultimately able to come out in the public sphere as writers and poets. Purnshashi Debi was fortunate to receive the support of her brother as well, and she graciously acknowledges that in *Mone Pare*. Learning to read and write were transgressions that symbolized women stepping out of the class, caste, and gender boundaries, which were believed to secure their purity and honor.

The support and encouragement of male members of the family, although important, did not mean freedom from domestic responsibilities. Unfortunately, at the tender age of 13, Debi became a mother only to lose the child within a matter of weeks. This incident left a deep imprint on her. Over the next few years, following the death of her child, Purnashashi Debi traveled to a number of places, including Kangra and Lahore. These travels not only gave her wonderment and joy, they also became the focus of her writings. There is an exhilarating description of her time in the Kangra Valley, which also seems to have revived her emotionally from the trauma she suffered after her child's death.

Her life continued to be very eventful with a lot of ups and downs. She published her first short story, *Abha*, which received an award from the Kuntaleen Press. She also lost her second child, who had developed pneumonia, and she too became seriously ill. Debi was taken to the Mari hills near Rawalpindi to her brother's home (her brother had purchased and used to run an English press) in the hope that the change of scenery would heal her physically and emotionally. Travels like these again became a source of inspiration for her writings. *Mone Pare* is filled with portrayals of nature, people, and Debi's own affective states as she visited new places.

However, these trips – to Kashi, which she later made her home, Nabha in Patiala, and Dehradun, were accompanied by a succession of deaths of intimate family members – her elder sister, sister-in-law, mother, and two daughters. Deaths in her immediate family were a ceaseless reality for Debi. As I mention earlier, her husband Pyarimohan passed away all of a sudden in 1932. Toward the end of her life she lost three of her adult sons in 1950, 1961, and 1964. Purnashashi is silent about these deaths, except in the last section of *Mone Pare*. Instead we get to know about her writings, her recognition in the literary field, and her work as the head mistress of a girls' school in Daltongan, presently in the state of Jharkhand. Debi also suffered from severe illnesses including a stroke that incapacitated her physically and intellectually for a few years.[54]

During these protracted bleak times the beauty and grace of nature gave her comfort. Purnashashi Debi's portrayal of nature's beauty in *Mone Pare* is a window to her broader affective life, which in turn found expression in her writing. These affective states, while expressing wonder and joy on seeing new places and at natural beauty, were often poignantly laced with the sorrow of losing so many loved ones throughout her adult life.

Apart from Debi's travels and the sorrows caused by the deaths of so many loved ones, her life as a widow, first in Vrindavan and then at Varanasi (Kashi), was a crucial element of her social and moral critique that also went to the heart of her ethic of care. Vrindavan was, and still is, a refuge for widowed women, who were outcasts in Hindu society and whose only hope of belonging lay at the feet of Lord Krishna. Debi's first encounter with Vrindavan is an affectively charged portrayal of the discrimination women faced without the economic and social protection of their husbands or any other male member of the family:

> Vrindavandhaam! I have always had a deep desire to come here, but I never dreamt it would be like this. What I never thought – being the playground of Radha and Krishna. Vrindavan is truly an abode of happiness. But how can one feel any pleasure when a fire is burning inside you? But for a wanderer who is exhausted from the hazards of travel, lost on a stormy night, being able to see a single star peering from the thick clouds is a great relief. Similarly for me, amidst the upheavals of my life, there was a flicker of hope in my heart – I wanted to devote the rest of my life to the service of the Lord who shelters everyone and forget all my pain. It is all *maya* [illusion]. The reason behind all this torture, disrespect, and suffering is *maya*.[55]

And then she poignantly added, 'I am unable to take any more pain'. She is silent on how the events which led her to express such intense emotions that had unfolded when she moved to Vrindavan.

This emotionally charged narrative, nevertheless, reflects the social consciousness that became visible in her literary creations. The kinship she felt with Krishna/Madhav/Shyam not only assuaged her physically and emotionally, but there is a sense of her being emancipated in and through her newfound faith.[56] It was again a male, albeit Lord Krishna, who seemed to have come to her support. But it would be wrong to read this as Debi giving in to male dominance or to religion. Faith and religion as a means to banish (widowed) women from society struck her as a particularly cruel custom of the upper caste Hindus and the patriarchal structure did not evade her criticism.

Her move from Vrindavan to Varanasi represented a stark contrast in the sense that she did not have to live in a community of widowed women, whose every act seemed a commemoration of their banishment. She writes about her memories of her first visit to the holy city of Kashi (Varanasi), as young bride. Being surrounded by family members, at that time she could witness the beauty of the city only superficially. When she visited the city for a longer period, as a widow, she could also see the filth and muck beneath the outward beauty. She was particularly struck by the deceit and falsehood that took place in one of the holiest Hindu sites. She was particularly pained at the plight of women.

The experiences of Shukhalata Rao, Priyabala Gupta, and Purnashashi Debi, the three women writers whose autobiographies and other writings I have examined in this chapter, although different, are reflective of the struggles that women faced in a gendered and patriarchal society. These women writers, in spite of the enormous difficulties they faced, effectively utilized their experiences to devise their ethics of care. In this chapter I have shown how discourses and practices of health and wellbeing cannot be abstracted from biographies of women in a gendered and patriarchal society. Nevertheless, it would be shortsighted to frame these experiences through simple binaries of colonial/Indian, subjugating/subjugated, public/private, and so on. My concern, apart from highlighting the hierarchical gendered context within which women lived, wrote, and practiced care, has been to highlight these women's complex and often contradictory and ambivalent articulations of beliefs and values.

5
Affective Remedies: Advertisements and Cultural Politics of Hygiene

Globally, in the late nineteenth and the early twentieth centuries, advertisements became a vital medium for the promotion of a range of commodities. 'The pictorial advertisement', David Ciarlo argues, 'formed a new world of "commercial visuality", which was simultaneously a business practice that drove unprecedented expansion of imagery across many different media, and a new and prominent cultural field', which dramatically changed the very look of nations (Ciarlo, 2011). Advertisements concerning hygiene and sanitation in colonial India/Bengal had a similar impact. India too was a part of this expanding 'commercial visuality'.

The late nineteenth and the first half of the twentieth centuries witnessed a surge of advertisements in commercial and popular culture. In fact, for the growing market of patent medicines, advertising in the popular press was the only cost effective way to reach a sizeable clientele. Advertisements of this period, which was a politically vibrant time in India, were often animatedly political in their tones. The political tenor of medical advertisements, specifically their suturing into the colonial context, however, gave commercial visuality in India a different texture.

This chapter discusses the relationship between nation, empire, and late nineteenth- and early twentieth-century commercial visual culture in India. It explores how advertisements for hygienic/beauty products framed and 'moved' debates on empire, nationhood, consumption, and cultural belonging in Bengal and India as a whole. Emotions/affect around ideas of empire, nation, class, and gender, as this chapter shows, were frequently utilized in advertisements to create a clientele for hygiene and beauty products. As such, these advertisements created particular sentiments around empire, nation, consumption, and wellbeing. 'Advertising's empire was built, in part, on the advertising of empire', as Ciarlo suggests.[1] Advertising was also effectively utilized by the Indian middle class to promote indigenous therapeutic systems and to further its own agendas.

My study focuses on late nineteenth- and early twentieth-century Bengali and English advertisements in newspapers and popular journals. Through an analysis of these advertisements, this chapter explores the development of the medical marketplace and medical consumerism in Bengal. In particular, it investigates four constitutive elements of this process, namely the commodification of hygiene, medical 'pluralism', the gendered nature of the new hygienic consciousness, and affects which animated the medical consumer commodity marketplace.

More broadly, in this chapter, I explore the following questions: What was the role of medical advertising in the chronicles of the history of medicine? To what extent can an understanding of the medical marketplace in India offer a new understanding of concepts such as hygiene, cleanliness, health, and wellbeing – concepts that remain central to discourses of preventive medicine? How were empire, nationalism, and the accompanying social, economic, and political changes entwined in the development of a medical marketplace? How was domesticity – as a site of ideological and practical intervention – used to create a group of potential consumers and practitioners, especially among middle class women and men? And how did enchantment affectively enable the ways in which these therapeutic and restorative advertisements became meaningful and acceptable?

In the first section, 'Enchantments of empire and nation', I explore the affective relationship between consumption and enchantment in the context of empire and nation. The second section, titled 'Advertisements, consumer culture, and empire', explores imperial entanglements of visual representations and advertisements. It excavates the colonial textures of medical and hygienic advertisements, particularly in their endorsements and stylistic particularities. In the third section, 'Advertisements in a pluralist medical marketplace', I explore the strikingly diffuse and fragmented nature of the colonial medical marketplace within which the authority of any one particular type of medicine (whether homeopathic, allopathic, or Ayurvedic) was far from complete. Finally, in the concluding section, 'Contagion of advertisements', I analyze the circuits of affect in and through which advertisements framed and, in turn, were legitimized by ideas of consumption and national belonging.

Enchantments of empire and nation

By the late nineteenth and the early twentieth centuries, advertisements were commercially and culturally thriving in Bengal and other parts of India. A surge in newspaper and other print media circulation and advancements in lithography and photography provided advertisers with fertile means to effectively endorse a wide variety of products and commodities that were flooding the market, and they seized this opportunity. Advertisements, with their images, messages, and stylistic adornments become a visual phenomenon that evoked both bewilderment and criticism. Yet although complaints about advertisements taking over the lives and desires of middle class women and men were common, these advertisements and the broader commercial visuality symbolized a magical urbanscape that was becoming common in colonial India. In short, medical advertising became a cultural experience beset with paradoxes. I describe the commercial visuality that simultaneously provoked marvel, wonderment, and objection, as a paradox of enchantment.

Enchantment seems to be making a comeback in scholarly narratives of modernity. One consequence of this shift is that disenchantment as the overarching condition of capitalist modernity is being questioned.[2] Michael Saler and Joshua Landy, for example, argue that if modernity and disenchantment have gone hand in hand, enchantment has been a parallel reality as well: 'The progressive disenchantment of the world was thus accompanied, from the start and continually, by its progressive re-enchantment.'[3] Questioning the commonly accepted narrative trope of modernity, Saler writes:

> In recent years historians from disparate fields have independently challenged the long-standing sociological view that modernity is characterized by 'disenchantment'. This view, in its broader terms, maintains that wonders and marvels have been demystified by

science, spirituality has been supplanted by secularism, spontaneity has been replaced by bureaucratization, and the imagination has been subordinated to instrumental reason.[4]

The emergent view that modernity is as enchanted as it is disenchanted may conjure alternative vistas to the historical imagination, and at the very least offers the possibility of pulling new rabbits out of old hats....[5]

While Saler agrees that disenchantment was a powerful reality, he also contends that parallel processes of enchantment have always been at work.

The myths and magic that have continued to persist despite the alienating iron grip of modernity have kept alive the possibilities for enchantment, argues Saurabh Dube.[6] For Dube, the same modernity that produced alienation and disenchantment also authored its own enchantments:

These extend from the immaculately imagined origins and ends of modernity through to the dense magic of money and markets; and from novel mythologies of nation and empire through to hierarchical oppositions between myth and history, emotion and reason, ritual and rationality, East and West, and tradition and modernity.[7]

What I find provocative and useful in Dube's argument is the degree of intimacy with which he defines the relationship between the enthralling and estranged sides of modernity. This intimate accord (even if it is in tension) between the two, according to Dube, has to be understood as productive co-existence, albeit strained. Moreover, the antinomies between disenchantment and enchantment with modernity need not be necessarily objectified or concretized. Rather, they could be thought of as frames, structures, conditions and possibilities for a range of happening and 'knowing' within diverse spaces and times. Empire, nation, and globalization are some of the sites where these antinomies are played out. Dube's work *Enchantments of Modernity* vouches for the 'magic' of modernity and presents it as that never-ending potentiality of state, market, myth, religion, and family, among others.[8]

Jane Bennett, on the other hand, defines enchantment as a 'mood' that signifies a 'pleasurable feeling of being charmed by the novel and as yet unprocessed encounter and...a more unheimlich [uncanny] feeling of being disrupted or torn out of one's default sensory-psychic–intellectual disposition'.[9] Thus, '[s]tarting from the assumption that the world has become neither inert nor devoid of surprise but continues to inspire deep and powerful attachments', she explores bases of modern political ethics:[10]

> My counterstory seeks to induce an experience of the contemporary world – a world of inequity, racism, pollution, poverty, violence of all kinds – as also enchanted – not a tale of reenchantment but one that calls attention to magical sites already here.[11]

Bennett analyzes commodities as an everyday site of enchantment. Bennett contends that although commodities are indeed 'enigmatic' and 'magical' objects, as Marxist scholars among others have convincingly shown, they, however, also possess a certain vitality that can be experienced as a genuine affective state. This affective state, according to Bennett, is similar to the experience of beauty that is sublime and lofty. Writing about a GAP advertisement called 'Khakis Swing' she provocatively claims: 'That style can be described as an aesthetic of vibrant mobility, of the ever-present possibility of bursts of vitality that violate an order ranking humans incomparably higher than animals, vegetables, and minerals.'[12]

My study of commercial visuality in colonial India draws on this scholarship on enchantments of modernity to open up a window into the complex and contested suturing of social, cultural, and political worlds in the making of a modern medical marketplace. While hygiene – as a modern discourse in colonial Bengal – was commonly couched in a language that emphasized crisis, degradation, and collapse, the fast growing marketplace sought to guarantee health, vitality, and cure for a range of common ailments. In this enchantment and disenchantment with modern hygiene, medical advertisements played a crucial role. These advertisements were tempting and appealing, not only because of the possibilities of cure they offered, but also because their 'visual' representation of a vast range of commodities was 'magical'. In order to historicize the affective vitality of commercial culture in the context of empire, in the next section, I will first map the linkages between consumer culture, advertising, and empire.

Advertising, consumer culture, and empire

Visuality was a vital dimension in the functioning of empire. Photographs, paintings, and maps, along with other visual techniques, became representational archives. These archives not only presented the cultural and political endeavors of the empire, they were also repositories of the desires and sensibilities that guided imperial projects. As such, to appropriate Martin Jay and Sumathy Ramaswamy's suggestion, these representational archives 'demonstrate that an appreciation of the role of visual experience is necessary for understanding the functioning of hegemonic imperial power and the ways that the colonized subjects spoke, and looked back at their imperial rulers'. Jay and Ramaswamy also argue that education in new systems of images and viewing highlights how such visual politics took place not just in the metropole of the empire, but in the peripheries as well.[13]

As with the representational politics of empire, commodities and consumer culture have constituted a productive site for understanding the economic, political, social, and cultural operations of empire. Scholarship on empires is now plush with explorations of the commodities, markets, commerce, and consumerism that were thriving in most empires by the middle of the nineteenth century. In fact, at one level, it is impossible to separate the deep entanglements of empire and commodity culture given that colonial and imperial projects started as commercial endeavors.

Scholars such as Thomas Richards, Anne McClintock, and Timothy Burke, among others, have offered some of the most provocative and thoughtful studies on empire's commodities, consuming cultures, and visual extravaganza. These scholars have explored the spectacle that commodity cultures had brought in to the imperial hotspots by the mid-nineteenth century. This period in history is commonly labeled an era of 'commodity capitalism' and, not surprisingly, advertising as an industry began in earnest around the same time. Richards, in his exploration of the rise of spectacle as a consumer, cultural, and political posture or mode in Victorian Britain, writes: 'It consisted primarily of a rhetorical mode of amplification and excess that came to pervade and structure public and private life in the nineteenth century, and it originated in the legitimation crisis that followed in the wake of the French Revolution and the Napoleonic Wars.'[14]

The spectacle was carried forward from the eighteenth century, but it acquired new attire. 'In a variety of ways nineteenth century consumers were witnessing the modulated transformation of the remnants of the high style into the basic tropes of a new commodity culture.' Spectacle, Richards further argues, was transformed into a 'new kind of political theater' that 'came at a time when the high style of representation had fallen into general disrepute'.[15] This emergent spectacle of commodification, however, had distinct imperial underpinning. Anne McClintock argues that the spectacular growth in the production and consumption of soaps from the late nineteenth century occurred as soap commercials were framed and popularized within a narrative of imperial prowess, gendered domesticity, and racism:

> In order to manage the great soap show, an aggressively entrepreneurial breed of advertisers emerged, dedicated to gracing each homely product with a radiant halo of imperial glamour and racial potency. The advertising agent, like the bureaucrat, played a vital role in the imperial expansion of foreign trade.[16]

Timothy Burke, similarly, has studied the imperial networks of commodity culture in colonial Zimbabwe that gave rise to an increasing demand for and consumption of soaps, creams, deodorants, and disinfectants. In *Lifebuoy Men, Lux Women*, Burke explains how this market for hygienic commodities in the context of Southern Africa utilized and produced powerful vocabularies about physicality, race, and civilization. He shows how white colonizers' understanding of black African bodies was deeply inflected by characterizations of physical unsanitariness and racial degeneracy. Cleanliness was highlighted as an index of civilizational greatness and African bodies were argued to be intrinsically inferior in this regard. Richards traces the history of this commodity culture, which, subsequently, was appropriated by Africans, much to the jubilation of colonial and African leaders and industrialists alike: 'The organizations, sentiments, and values that had been produced in this (hygiene and domesticity) field and the interlocking of various powers around bodily practice, manners, and identity all became increasingly commodified in the postwar era.'[17]

Spectacles of advertisements are thus an important site for understanding the cultural production of empires and nations at the intersections of class and gender. It is also important to highlight the limits of this spectacular co-production of empire and advertising. In the context of Bengal, for example, as I show in the next section, the medical marketplace became a contested space for a range of therapeutic systems and products and it did not present unequivocal dominance of allopathic (read European medical) ideas and products.

Advertisements and a pluralist medical marketplace

The medical marketplace in colonial Bengal operated on a simple principle – supply of a variety of therapies for a variety of maladies.[18] This principle was strengthened because of the regeneration of several already existing therapeutic systems in late nineteenth- and early twentieth-century Bengal and India as a whole. Ayurveda, for example, was given fresh impetus by enthusiasts such as Gangaprasad Sen, Neelamber Sen, and Gangadhar Ray, who were inspired to establish the N.N. Sen and Company Private Limited to undertake large scale production of pharmaceuticals. Ayurvedic drugs were commercialized also because of the efforts of other companies such as Dhaka Oushadhalaya, Sadhana Oushadhalaya, and Kalpataru Ayurvedic Works.[19] Homeopathy was another system of medicine that became immensely popular in urban Bengal.[20] David Arnold and Sumit Sarkar argue that homeopathic treatment found increasing favor among urban Bengalis because it was cheap, easy to use, and not associated with British colonial authority.[21] The monopoly of allopathic drugs was therefore far from complete.[22]

Another factor that crucially impacted on the Indian market was the disruption caused by World War I, which led to a drastic decline in imports and, consequently, a growth in local production of therapeutic drugs and hygienic products. Many of these commercial undertakings also had nationalist underpinnings. For example, the Bengal Chemicals and Pharmaceutical Works Limited, which was established in 1901 through the pioneering efforts of Acharya Prafulla

Chandra Ray, became the first drug factory that was completely owned and managed by Indians.

The plurality of the medical marketplace was starkly evident in the advertisements of the period. Newspapers, popular journals, and magazines advertised a wide variety of cures and therapies for a range of ailments. These advertisements present an extremely important site to explore the negotiations of a host of material as well as the epistemological issues that were crucial in charting the contours of medical practice in late colonial India. While semantically dense and culturally meaningful in their own right, in colonial India, these advertisements were also a part of a broader milieu that bridged the political practices of the state, the household, and the civil society.

By the 1880s, medical advertisements occupied a prominent place in newspapers. Such a dramatic increase in medical advertising led a writer in *Chikitsa Sammilani* ('A Compendium on Therapeutics', a popular medical journal in Bengali) to comment that the number of advertisements for allopathic, homeopathic, *hakimi*, Ayurvedic, and 'patent' medicines paralleled the number of diseases in India.[23] This remark was not unfounded, because by the early 1900s, advertisements for medicines, hygienic products, and 'miraculous remedies' consumed more than fifty percent of advertising space in Indian newspapers.[24] Ointments, eye drops, pills for all kinds of ailments, and Ayurvedic medicines for the cure of nerve diseases, asthma, and 'weaknesses' were regularly advertised items.

This pluralist medical marketplace, to a certain extent, was a result of colonial policies. Anil Kumar argues that pharmacology did not take off in India until the early twentieth century because of a sustained 'drug import' policy by the British government. Consequently, a thriving universe of 'bazaar drugs' emerged in the late nineteenth and early twentieth centuries.[25] Many newspapers of the time devoted several pages to advertising, and advertisements for medical cures and therapies constituted an important focus of those pages. A page from the English newspaper *The Indian Mirror*, from 1889, illustrates the competitive field of medical advertising very well: at least five advertisements pertained to different cures for painful menstruation, syphilis, cholera, and diseases of the liver, stomach, kidney, and bowels. And alongside them were advertisements for baby care products such as Cuticura skincare remedies.[26]

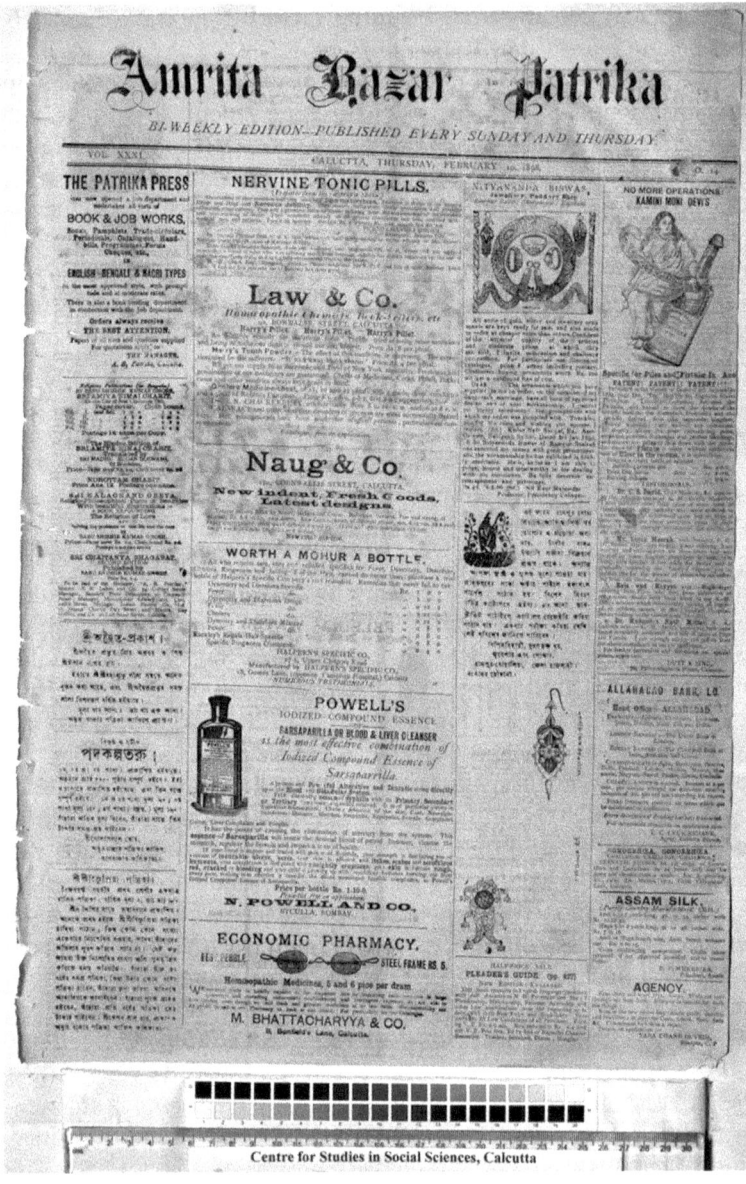

Figure 5.1 Page of a newspaper from 1898 showing the advertisements of medical products from a variety of medical knowledge systems *Amrita Bazar Patrika*, February 10, 1898

Holloway Pills, 'The Great Indian Remedy for Cholera', Dr B.M. Sircar's Abroma Augustum for painful menstruation, Paul & Co.'s Proprietary Medicines, the 'wonderful medicine' – Beecham's Pills, and Hakim Najut Ali Shah Kadiri's prescription for a wide variety of conditions, to name a few, together presented a 'visual' landscape of advertisements that showcased medical pluralism in colonial Bengal. The visual landscape of medical advertising was, however, of a limited nature, particularly in its limited use of images and pictures. Most advertisements were linguistic statements with some information about the composition of advertised drugs and concoctions. They also often included testimonials from users happily endorsing the products.[27]

It is relevant to note that the birth of 'modern' newspapers in India also marked the emergence of advertising. James Hicky, a surgeon by profession and a disgruntled employee of the East India Company, owned the *Bengal Gazette*, often touted as the first newspaper in India. The *Bengal Gazette* started publication in 1780, but its life was cut short by East India Company officials (particularly Warren Hastings) who were unhappy with the candid reports that Hicky published on the corruption and misrule of Fort William.[28] In its brief period of circulation (1780–1782), the *Bengal Gazette* also carried advertisements, which were added by Hicky purely for monetary reasons. Medical advertisements in the newspaper were, however, mostly for 'patent' medicines – concoctions made by 'doctors' that were owned by and sold under their names. Indians joined commercial advertising much later, in 1905, when B. Dattaram & Company was set up for this purpose.

The early twentieth century also marked a shift in the representational style and tone of newspaper advertisements. A significant reason for this change was the emergent anti-colonial struggle and the high-handed British response to newspapers. A case in point was the *Amrita Bazar Patrika*. Published originally in Bengali by Tusharkanti Ghose and his father Sisir Kumar Ghose, *Amrita Bazar Patrika* became the target of the British government's wrath for its support of India's freedom movement. In 1878 *Amrita Bazar Patrika* was converted into an English daily to escape the draconian Vernacular Press Act.

Parallel to the growing engagement of newspapers in the political dialogues of the late nineteenth and early twentieth centuries, advertising became front and central to newspapers' business. This shift in advertising tactic was in fact quite literal. In an October 1905 edition of the *Amrita Bazaar Patrika*, for example, the front page was crowded with advertisements. Advertisements for drugs and other medical products constituted a significant percentage of such front-page coverage. 'Powell's Essence of Sarsaparilla or Blood and Liver Cleanser', 'Pandit Gopalachary's Ayurvedic Plague Remedies', 'B. Laughliin's & Co, Chemist's Healing Balm', and 'Bharat Vaisajyanilaya's Vigor Pills' were some of the prominently advertised items.

In addition to highlighting the competitive and pluralistic medical marketplace of colonial Bengal, these advertisements also exhibited a range of cultural tropes. In the advertisement for 'Bharat Vaisajyanilaya's Vigor Pills', for example, efficacy was assured by '[t]hat Renowned Swami Dharmananda Mahabharati'.[29] This concoction, which claimed to be an effective cure for 'physical lassitude', 'nervous debility', and 'wasting diseases' boasted of an exclusive Hindu Ayurvedic pharmacopoeia, whose value was often certified by a Hindu religious leader. Such interweaving of religious and national imaginaries with claims of pharmacological efficacy was quite common in the advertisements of that period.

The Swadeshi movement and the resultant politically charged anti-colonial climate of the early twentieth century also found expression in the advertisements. The rhetorical style of these advertisements not only emphasized what Madhuri Sharma calls the 'codes of local culture', these advertisements were also surrounded by news and announcements with politically explicit language supporting Swadeshi and boycott to give them a distinct political flavor. Deployment of particular cultural and political tropes was also directed at gaining market control. 'The Indian drug manufacturers of allopathic or indigenous medicine', Sharma argues, 'tried various methods to tighten their grip on Indian consumers'.[30] Evocative phrases such as 'Your Blood Is Calling for Help' for an advertisement for Clarke's Blood Mixture, or 'Don't Be in the Dark' for the 'most marvelous cure for Rheumatism' were common in medical advertisements in the newspapers.[31]

Until the turn of the twentieth century, as discussed earlier, advertisements hardly included any images or photographs, which, however, began to change soon thereafter. But even then the images were pretty minimalist in their techniques and scope. A full-page advertisement for Kabiraj K.L. Roy's Ayurvedic remedies in *Amrita Bazar*

Patrika in 1923, for example, had no images. The advertisement asked in bold letters, 'Have You Tried Our Medicine?', and thereafter presented a detailed description of each of the drugs manufactured by the drug company and the specific ailments each of them targeted. Images thus remained secondary to the elaborate printed text that supplied specific information about particular remedies and their manufacturers.[32]

Although newspaper advertisements witnessed significant growth in the postwar period, when Indian markets were inundated with foreign goods, advertising did not become a specialized profession until the 1930s. The first Indian owned advertising agency, the National Advertising Agency, was established in 1931. Realizing the potential of advertising, newspapers started carrying testimonials that reiterated its importance. In 1932, the well-known newspaper *Bengalee*, for example, carried a notice: 'Proof That It Pays To Advertise'.[33] This was a testimony by the Advertising Association's Research Department, which claimed that bold advertising by companies even in times of depression could maintain or even increase profits. Such testimonials for advertising were not uncommon. Another one stated: 'Put Your Faith in an Advertised Good'.[34] Professional advertising added another twist to visual commercial culture. However, advertising continued to mark a pluralist medical marketplace.

Advertising in colonial Bengal commodified not only medical and hygienic products, but also, as I have been showing, medical ideologies. That is to say, advertisements presented not only competing medicinal products, but also medical ideologies. The way in which medicines and healthcare products 'representing' different medical systems were advertised together was particularly striking.[35] The *Statesman*, for example, had advertisements eulogizing *hakimi* treatments, homeopathy, and surgical dentistry on the same page. Similarly, *Amrita Bazar Patrika* regularly advertised 'genuine ayurvedic medicines' along with, for example, the magic touch of 'germolene', which, at that time, was a commonly used medicine in many parts of the British Empire.

Advertisements in newspapers, and also in popular magazines and journals, offered a richly diverse world of therapeutic and hygienic commodities and products. These advertisements, apart from representing a distinctly pluralistic medical marketplace, also created and transformed a consumer class in late colonial India. They also become an important site for the expression of medical ideologies, vocabularies, and rationalities that were implicated in drawing upon and further entrenching certain social hierarchies. Advertising of medical and hygienic products was, for example, deeply gendered. And this hierarchized gendering was, as I show in the following, most starkly evident in advertisements for hygiene and cosmetic products.

Advertising beauty, womanhood, and domesticity

Soaps, talcum powder, hair oil, facial, dental, and shaving creams, and a variety of essences and perfumes constituted a popular range of cosmetics that were advertised as hygienic products in colonial Bengal. The focus of medicine on personal cleanliness and hygiene in the early twentieth century led to soaps and dental creams being frequently advertised as medicinal items.

Personal cleanliness and hygiene had wide scope and encompassed a range of domains and concerns. Under the label of hygiene and cleanliness, cures for ocular and dental ailments, common coughs and colds, weakness and frailty, fevers, a wide variety of stomach ailments, rheumatism and arthritis, and women's reproductive health related problems, especially menstrual dysfunctions, were commonly advertised. The scope of health and hygiene was even wider. Baby food (primarily formula milk), one of the most advertised items during the early years of the twentieth century, was framed as a health and hygiene product. And health products for building physical strength, such as barley, special foods, and tonics also fell within this category.

Apart from newspapers, which were common sites for medical advertisements as discussed earlier, popular magazines constituted another important venue for the advertisement of the wide range of health and hygiene products. For example, *Chikitsha Sammilani*, a magazine that had the explicit goal of bringing together discussions on allopathic, homeopathic, and *kabiraji* systems of medicine, used to have a regular section on 'Deshiye Swasthye Roop or Jouban' (Secrets of Beauty and Youth in Indigenous Medicine). Entries in this section, emphasizing the need for the right mix of physical and emotional comportment for ideal health, presented discussions on longevity, countenance, and beauty. Writers frequently complained about premature graying of hair, weak eyesight, poor dental hygiene, and skin diseases among the youth and highlighted the perceived inter-linkages between health, hygiene, ability, and beauty.[36]

Grihasthamangal (Welfare of the Household) was another Bengali magazine that discussed and advertised beauty and hygienic products. In 1927, it had started as an agricultural guidebook with information on farming, the use of pesticides, manures, etc. It also published articles on trade and commerce, public health, medicine, domestic science, and women's issues.[37] Advertisements in *Grihasthamangal* were illustrative of the range of products that were brought together under the rubric of beauty and personal hygiene: an essence called Mandar, which was described as 'heavenly in its fragrance', scented til (sesame seed) hair oil, Chawanprash – a health tonic from Bengal Chemicals, hair dye, hair removing cream, Cutona for skin disorders, 'parijat snow', and Jabakusum Hair Oil.[38]

Several of these products explicitly drew together medicinal and cosmetic benefits and had a gendered target audience. Jabakusum Hair Oil, one such product, was a very popular hair tonic/oil in Bengal. Calcutta-based C.K. Sen & Company, which manufactured this oil, claimed to use Ayurvedic ingredients in its commercial cosmetic products. The gendered inflection is clearly visible in the advertisements for the oil. One version of this advertisement portrays an Indian woman sitting inside the open petals of a huge hibiscus flower, which was the main ingredient of the product. Clothed in a sari, the lady holds a bottle of Jabakusum Hair Oil and the caption reads: 'The softness of flowers in my hair'. The advertisement further reiterates: 'Jabakusum makes it possible'.[39]

Gendered representations of hygienic-beauty products were not unusual. In the early twentieth century, advertisements in Bengal (and in other parts of India) deployed women and family as important sites for the production of a new consumer ethos. And domesticity provided the broader ideology to justify this ethos. In this regard colonial Bengal was no different from other parts of the world and, in a significant way, it also highlights genealogical links to postcolonial deployments of domesticity in hygiene. Timothy Burke, for example, shows how in 'modern' Zimbabwe hygiene – as a powerful set of social, economic, and cultural practices – was framed through gendered constructions of African domesticity and of women's roles as wives and mothers. Colonial missionary discourse, African and English newspapers and the popular press, business

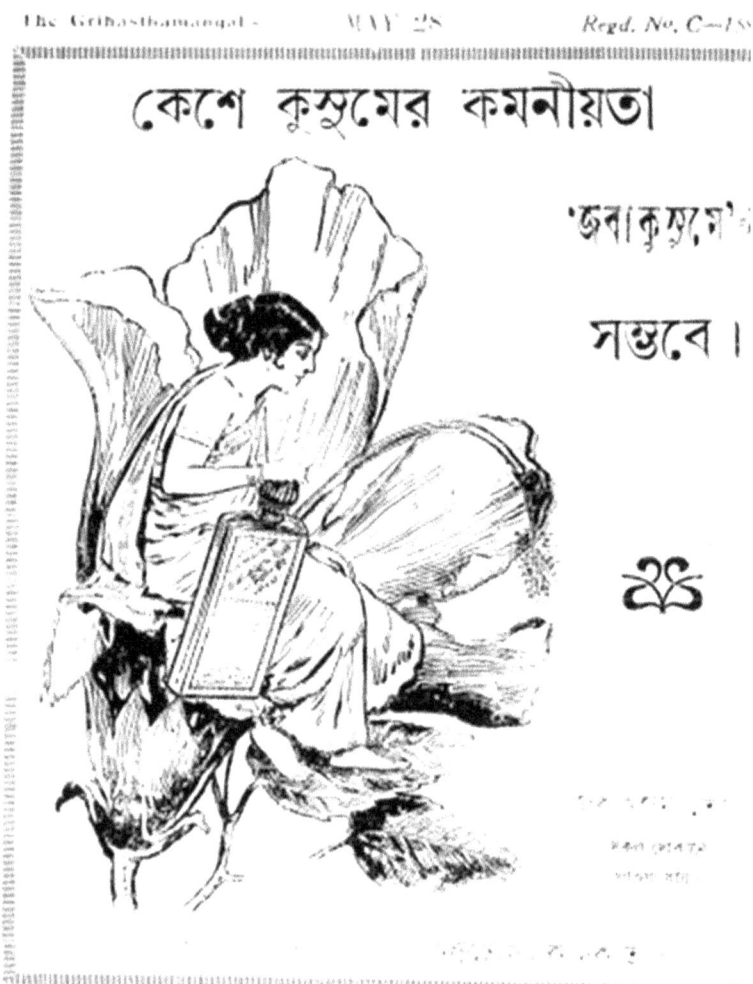

Figure 5.2 Advertisement of Jabakusum Hair Oil from *Grihasthamangal*, May 28, 1928

organizations, and colonial state activities converged on what they considered the single most important role of wives and mothers as agents and practitioners of modern hygiene. Not surprisingly, as *Lifebuoy Men, Lux Women* shows, advertising played a crucial role in preaching and popularizing hygiene and its gendered constructions in colonial and postcolonial Zimbabwe.[40]

Bengali advertisements for beauty and hygienic products were similarly framed within the domain of the *grihastha/paribar* (household/domestic) realm through the figure of the wife and mother. Domesticity, although it continued to have central focus in the advertising of beauty and hygienic products, was portrayed somewhat differently from the first decade of the twentieth century. Advertisements started to use images of Indian women to endorse beauty products and words such as 'beauty' or 'charm' were commonly deployed with reference to Indian women.

In contrast, advertisements until the turn of the twentieth century showed slim British/Western women attired in what were considered to be less decorous clothes; they also often depicted women who seemed to have stepped into the public realm. This was particularly ironic because some of these advertisements, such as those for fairness creams, specially targeted Bengali and other Indian women, urging them to use these creams in order to become fairer like their European counterparts. Nevertheless, the 'femininity' conferred on Bengali women in these advertisements always referred to the 'woman within her household'.[41] By the 1920s, however, deployment of images of Indian women was common in advertisements for beauty and hygienic products such as soaps, hair oils, and perfumes.[42]

These advertisements involving Bengali women fundamentally targeted motherhood and presented the figure of the woman almost exclusively as a mother. The advertisements for health and hygiene commodities during this period marked a continuity with the earlier era (between the 1890s and early 1900s) in depicting hierarchically gendered constructions of the medical profession – male physicians were shown to have the expertise in and by themselves, even for the diseases of women and children, while women, if they were shown, were often portrayed as certificate holding midwives.[43] I will come back to this point later in this chapter. At present I wish to focus on the porous boundary and symbiotic relationship between health and beauty products.

Apart from magazines and women's journals, newspapers constituted another important site for advertisements for beauty/health/ hygiene products. In the following I focus particularly on advertisements for soaps and hair oils in Indian and British owned newspapers. Soaps like Pears, Lux, and Sunlight were aggressively marketed and were much in demand. Pears soap, one of the oldest soap brands in the world, was an important tool – with its own contagious effects – in Britain's imperial project and its zeal to stamp out the physical and moral uncleanliness of African and Asian bodies.

Pears soap was first introduced to the Indian market in 1902 by A.F. Pears, and later it was manufactured and marketed by the Lever Brothers. Pears soap advertisements were common in Indian newspapers, particularly in the English language ones. Women constituted the dominant icons of Pears soap's colonial period advertisements and their images were used to depict the gendered nature of soap consumption. Not unlike other advertisements, in the early years of its introduction, advertising of Pears soap too utilized images of European women at first and later shifted to those of Indian women. In the early twentieth century, Pears advertisements consisted of drawings of faces of Indian women wearing a bindi (colored dot on the forehead) with the Pears soap in a wrapper at the bottom of the page and captions such as 'Protect Such Loveliness' or 'Keep your Skin Young'. These advertisements, which were mostly black and white representations, also consisted of detailed descriptions of the way in which the soap was supposed to work on not just the skin, but also feelings. They thereafter proclaimed: 'Make Pears Soap your daily beauty ritual'.

Later, around the mid-twentieth century, Pears soap advertisements sought to highlight the 'Indian'. One such advertisement consisted of a colored painting of a Hindu female deity holding a child and sitting inside the open petals of a lotus flower. The deity is adorned with a red and golden saree and is covered from head to foot in jewels, including a gold mace in her right hand. She sits in a manner that resembles the usual depictions of the goddess Lakshmi seated on the lotus flower with her consort Lord Vishnu. In this advertisement, however, the 'goddess' is shown as a caring mother who vouches for the purity of Pears soap. The advertisement is captioned – 'Pure as the Lotus' – and is accompanied with the statement: 'Learn without Sorrow the Eternal Truth that Youth is Godlike and Beauty is Youth'. It is as though the enchantment of consumer culture had to be supported by the gods, particularly when it came to the colonies.

The advertisements for Sunlight soap were similarly evocative and they too often drew upon distinctly religious iconography. Images of gods and goddesses from the Hindu pantheon, either in black and white or color, testified to the 'purity' of Sunlight soaps. A blue colored Vishnu sits on his mount, the Garuda, with the goddess Lakshmi by his side, as this picture of the advertisement shows, as a guarantor of Sunlight Soaps' 'pinnacle of purity'.

The representational styles of newspaper advertisements were not uniform. There were variations, particularly dependent upon ownership, i.e. whether they were British/European or Indian manufactured products. Advertisements for European owned health and beauty products were replete with claims of 'purity', 'grace', being 'natural', and offering 'improvement'. The advertisements for soap, for example, commonly claimed to provide the 'purest' of beauty care. They also assured a step toward 'refinement' and the joy of 'existence'.[44] These advertisements, very similar to what Colin Campbell describes as the Other Ethic, claimed to pave the way for improvement of the self through certain acts of consumption. These advertisements actively portrayed pleasures that were predicted to satisfy both the body and the mind and encourage a higher sensation. Though the connection between body and soul was not directly shown, advertisements for products that were aimed at betterment of the body often linked it to the movement of the 'soul' to a higher level or ideal.

Advertisements for Indian products, in contrast, brought together the religious and the secular quite differently in their representations. Even at the height of anti-colonial nationalism, advertisements for Indian products did not display any direct connection between bodily pleasure and spiritual vitality. When gods and goddesses were used to highlight the purity (quality) of a product, it was most often to vouch for its authenticity and Indianness. That is, advertising of Indian products tried to motivate consumers by Indianizing the appeal. Advertisements by Bengal Chemical, Dhariwal, a woolen cloth dealer, The Hindu Biscuit Company, the Indian Homeopathic Laboratory, and Sakti Oushadhalaya, for example, emphasized the superior quality of Indian products.

Similarly, advertisements for Kuntaline – a perfumed oil that was frequently presented as being recommended by prominent personalities – vouched for its superior, Indian quality. This worldly orientation of advertisements for Indian products, even when spiritual language and figures were utilized, was significant also because the vocabulary of anti-colonial cultural nationalism continually emphasized upper caste Hindu spirituality. That is, even when they were Indianized and/or guaranteed by spiritual leaders, these goods explored a world of everyday consumption largely as a new and powerful reality of the domestic household and the nation.

The medical marketplace in late colonial Bengal had a mutually productive relationship with the Bengali household. New courses of domestic consumption were being charted by the medical marketplace, which, at the same time, were emerging as a result of shifting imperatives of the domestic. In these mutual transformations of the domestic and medical marketplaces, women were commonly projected as agents for change in the habits of the family, particularly in relation to food. Hygiene and health were shown as tools that women could, and should, wield through the food they chose for their families.

Patented health foods occupied an important place in these household targeted advertisements. The entry of products such as Robinson's Barley, Cadbury's Cocoa, Brown and Polson's Corn Flour, Nestlé's Swiss Milk Chocolate, Ovaltine, and Malted Milk into the Indian market gave birth to a new vocabulary for securing health and vitality.[45] The striking aspect of this discourse on 'vitalism' was the way in which these advertisements combined an ideal of the 'naturalness' and 'purity' of one place to the lack of the same in another, namely the 'hot climate of India'. Jackson Lears labels this commonly used trope 'imperial primitivism'.[46]

'Cadbury's Cocoa was made in an English factory in a Garden Village amidst pure and healthful surroundings', 'Liptons's Jams and Fruits [were] better than all others because Lipton [used] only English Grown Fruit', and 'Ovaltine was from Britain's most fertile fields and richest pastures'.[47] Such references to the English or British origins of the commodities were used as a guarantee of the genuineness, purity, and superiority of those products. Mechanization of the process further enhanced these qualities. Hence advertisements for formula baby milk were typically labeled 'completely untouched by hand'. Such assurances added another layer of colonial reference by claiming that such foods were perfectly suitable for 'hot countries with hot climates'.

Advertisements for baby products presented not only imperial but also gendered constructions. They were typical in the invocation of the caring figure of the Bengali or Indian mother. In advertisements for baby tonics, baby foods, medications for children's ailments, and even Ayurvedic medications that promised to make 'women fertile and bless them with children' there was a definite affective strategy – the deployment of mother–child bonding to invoke a special connection with the consumer product. Such representations typically showed an Indian mother holding a child on her lap, draped in a saree, her head covered, and in postures that exemplified the Bengali and/or Indian cultural repertoire. In fact, as I showed earlier, even when a goddess was deployed in these advertisements, she had to be incarnated as a mother with a child.

Class and caste were other constitutive elements of the advertisements. Robert Goldman argues that advertisements appropriate and construct class in subtle ways rather than directly highlighting it.[48] One can make a similar observation with regard to advertisements in colonial Bengal, particularly in the early twentieth century. There were no overt references to class/caste in these advertisements. However, since hygienic and sanitary reform was a distinctly middle class agenda, advertisements portrayed that class' concerns as well. In most of the advertisements class was constructed by signifying activities, values, and social roles through a particular vocabulary. Words such as purity and quality not only had colonial underpinning, they were also commonly used to represent middle class notions of wellbeing. These representations were, as discussed earlier, gendered. Although images of women were commonly deployed to invoke middle class values, these advertisements did not portray middle class women as public beings until well into the middle of the twentieth century. This absence is striking given that by the early twentieth-century middle class women were increasingly entering professions and partaking in politics and social welfare in the public domain.

Contagion of advertisements

In *Sentimental Figures of Empire in Eighteenth-Century Britain and France*, Lynn Festa explores the 'sentimental mode' that guided the popular imagination in Britain and France. Festa argues that this rhetorical trope enabled the preservation of a sense of European self 'that knitted subject and object together in ways that were difficult to disentangle'. The power of the sentimental mode came from its ability to act as a 'form of social and cultural differentiation'.[49] She links the production of sentimentality as a literary trope with the rising dominion of the British and French empires. 'In distinguishing between subjects and objects of feeling', she writes, 'the sentimental seeks to define what is proper to the self and what can be shared by or exchanged with others: it polices the division of self from the world'.[50]

The domain of advertisements in late colonial Bengal defined and crystalized a deeply affective mode that was too engaged in policing 'the division of self from the world'. However, in the context of colonial Bengal, as I have shown, a number of selves and worlds collided – of the colonial and colonized, European and non-European, civilized and uncivilized, Indian and non-Indian/foreign, middle class and the rest, and so on.

Advertisements – through words and images – cumulatively evoked deep sentiments among people. There was a distinct sense of people being moved by this exploding visual realm of advertisements that found expression in various forms of writings and representations of the time. Many such expressions were critical of the emerging commodity culture, which, it was argued, eclipsed more profound values that should ideally guide individual and collective living. But, simultaneously, there was also a sense of marvel and wonder evident in the writings and advertisements of this period. Advertisements, drawing upon a thriving print culture in the form of newspapers, popular journals, and magazines, presented a marketplace flooded with a dizzying range of commodities by the early years of the twentieth century. The sheer variety of products and commodities and their enchanting representations of consumer desires made it impossible for people not to feel a certain sense of awe and enchantment. This affective realm, as its spectacular growth and impact testify, was definitely contagious.

In this chapter I have explored how contagion as a medical, economic, social, and cultural idea and practice was integral in the emergence of commercial visuality in colonial Bengal. Contagion had multiple meanings and was evoked through a wide variety of modes and contexts. In the medical marketplace a variety of commodities – drugs, concoctions, and hygienic/beauty products – addressed the anxieties that were produced by epidemics such as cholera and plague. Medical ideas like cleanliness and sanitation gained unprecedented urgency in the context of epidemics. Contagion also implied another kind of transmission – of a seemingly endless list of novel and chronic medical conditions (the fallout of a fast-paced and modern urban life), which were argued to plague middle class Bengalis or Indians. Dyspepsia, ailments of the nervous system, lack of vitality or energy, and blood related disorders were continually presented as 'contagions' that collectively inflicted the body of the nation and the society.

In the broader context of medical and hygienic anxieties and concerns, advertisements became central not only to representations of contagion as a set of ideas, commodities, and practice, but also to expanding their affective and practical impact. Contagion as a modern medical sensibility enabled advertisements – as a commercial and popular genre – to build and represent connections between objects, bodies, people, institutions, and events. In short, these advertisements were powerful media for cultural 'world making'.[51] Advertisements offered textual spaces or 'surfaces' that enabled certain emotions like enchantment, pleasure, vigor, and wellbeing to become the markers of class, national, and gendered belonging.

Advertisements made particular affects like enchantment and vitality appropriate and timely by authorizing their creation and circulation within particular social and cultural collectivities. Advertisements and the broader commercial visual culture in late colonial Bengal in their own unique ways debated some of the most charged political, economic, and cultural issues of the time. Advertisements thus constituted a crucial site to decipher how the 'subjects' and 'objects' of these important concerns were affectively produced and enacted.[52] Middle class women, for example, became one of the principal targets and agents in the advertising of health and hygienic products and in the process they became the subjects and objects of a range of issues pertaining to the nation, empire, and household.

Gender was expressed in and through 'purposes', 'problems', 'issues', and 'places' that were defined as being the exclusive and naturalized concerns of women.[53] Hygiene, health, and vigor became agendas to be lived, practiced, and consumed through women's activities thereby making those activities synonymous with homemaking, consuming, and nation building. Health and hygiene agendas were produced as ideologies in and through the deployment of the gendered responsibilities of women. Nevertheless, it is noteworthy that advertisements using women's images were not in circulation until the early years of the twentieth century.

Health, hygiene, vitality and salubriousness gained currency and particular intent through the discourses of public health. These were, however, not simply medical concerns. They simultaneously became cultural and social sensibilities and political ideals that were passionately discussed in the public realm. Hygiene was a charged feeling/sensibility as well. In late nineteenth- and early twentieth-century colonial India, hygiene became an anchoring point around which concerns about the vitality of the Indian political, economic, social, and cultural body coalesced. And advertising, and the attendant commercial visuality, was without a doubt a crucial site in the enactment of these concerns.

Conclusion

In 1894, in an article in a well-known Bengali medical journal, *Chikitsa Sammilani*, the author recounted a story of the goddess of cholera's visit to a village:

> One night as a saint sat under a tree deep in meditation he heard a lone woman entering the village. Surprised at the sight of a woman all by herself so late at night the saint asked her who she was. The woman said that she was the goddess of cholera and that she was heading to the village to end the lives of three men who resided there. The pious man told her to be extremely cautious so that she did not end up killing anyone else in that village. The cholera goddess assured him. But instead of three, three hundred villagers died during the visitation. As she was leaving the village the saint confronted her and expressed his anger at the goddess for failing to keep her promise. The goddess responded that she had only extinguished three lives; the remaining two hundred and ninety seven lives were lost because they were too fearful.[1]

The writer ended the essay with the recommendation that while panicking unnecessarily during a cholera outbreak might not be helpful, unqualified gallantry is foolhardy as well. He also reiterated the importance of emotional tranquility and cheerfulness even when an epidemic is ravaging the village. The more a person gives in to negative emotions like fear, grief, sadness, and anger, the author suggests, the stronger will be the assault of the disease on him or her.[2]

Contagion, as the essay above vividly illustrates, acts and spreads through *feeling*. Feeling is not merely an additive to pathogenic contact. It is integral to pathogenic action. Prescriptions for emotional and physical wellbeing for individual and collective bodies were common in popular writings on health, medicine, and hygiene in the second half of the nineteenth and early twentieth centuries. It was commonly argued that certain affects could worsen afflictions, while others had the power to check the spread of disease.

In *Contagions of Feeling* I have argued that affects are intrinsic to chronicles of health, hygiene, and wellbeing. Affect or emotion is a powerful site to study trajectories of contagion. Myths, metaphors, rhetoric, and conventions that make disease, health, and medicine socially and culturally meaningful also critically impact on the unfolding of epidemics. Articulations of affect may vary across societies and through history. Nonetheless, their profound impact cannot be ignored. Recently, an article in *The New York Review of Books* aptly titled 'Ebola in Liberia: An Epidemic of Rumors' showed how the unexpectedly high number of Ebola related deaths in Liberia were a result of political rumors.[3]

As Alison Bashford and Claire Hooker argue, contagion first and foremost is about contact.[4] Contagion, and its articulation through a diverse set of 'signifiers', implies contact and assurances or fears associated with contact and proximity. Bashford and Hooker list some of these signifiers – 'resistance,' 'immunity,' 'colonization,' 'hygiene,' 'blood,' 'plague,' and 'hysteria.' *Contagions of Feeling* shows how some of these signifiers are articulated in narratives of contact in the histories of disease and medicine in India. Specifically, it studies contacts and intimacies of ideas, emotions, objects/commodities, and people in late nineteenth- and early twentieth-century Bengal. It explores how each of these were defined, manipulated, and appropriated culturally, politically, and socially in the production of narratives of contagion.

In late nineteenth and early twentieth centuries Bengal, contagion simultaneously implied medical ideologies, political goals, social organization, and cultural metaphors. Contagion in medicine implied a diseased state that spread from one person to another. It also enfolded an anxiety – apprehension about the possibility of escalation – that often provided the impetus for divergent political goals. Moreover, contagion also constituted a set of sensibilities – cultural and social – that impacted not only on the emergence and intensification of disease, but also on the appropriation and creation of social hierarchies. Anxiety about contact and proximity were used, as I show in the book, to define the moral elitism of certain groups and institutions and thereby to justify and maintain social boundaries, in particular those of class, gender, caste, and nation. These social boundaries were woven into the cultural fabric in subtle ways, in stark contrast to the more severe boundary making in times of epidemiological or political crisis.

Women's autobiographical writings emphasized the affective contact across medicine and society and private and public. While writing about contagions of health and wellbeing, female authors did not fail to highlight the contagions of a patriarchal society that disrupted and appropriated women's lives and desires. These authors brought together experiences of places and things, desires of womanhood, and physical and spiritual growth in personal journeys to create their own ethic of care. These writings, musings, and reminiscences were contagion themselves. On the one hand, they created an affective community around a spiritual–moral feminism and on the other they highlighted and circulated sources and agents of social malaise, particularly those of class, caste, and religion.

Another domain that acted as contagion, while it created powerful visual representations of cures for diseases, special foods and tonics, and beauty products was that of advertisements. Advertisements for health and hygiene products enchanted and inspired awe and were pivotal in creating a commercial visual culture. They brought together commodities, images, and assurances to enable ideas and practices of consumption in colonial Bengal. Advertisements legitimized therapies, secured commerce, and created the own legitimacy within a rapidly evolving culture of commodities and consumption.

Personal narratives, advertisements, paintings, and films, along with medical and administrative records of health and hygiene, did not simply provide representations of contagion; they were contagions themselves. In colonial and postcolonial histories of the Indian nation food, hunger, health, and hygiene have not only been economically and politically pivotal, but also affectively compelling – stirring and pushing narratives of identity, belonging, life, and death.

Chittaprosad's *Hungry Bengal*, for example, still moves the nation to relive the poignant calamity of the Bengal Famine. Such postcolonial commemorations mockingly evoke the contagions of economic gluttony and political hypocrisies. And in the process they affectively connect colonial and postcolonial India.

Notes

1 Introduction: Contagion and Cultural Politics of Hygiene

1. Preston R. (1995) *The Hot Zone: The Terrifying True Story of the Origins of the Ebola Virus*, New York: New York Anchor. Garrett L. (1995) *The Coming Plague: Newly Emerging Diseases in a World Out of Balance*, New York: Penguin Group. Garrett L. (2001) *Betrayal of Trust: The Collapse of Global Public Health*, New York: Hachette Books.
2. India PHFI. About PHFI. Available at: https://www.phfi.org/about-us/about-phfi.
3. Ibid.
4. General Pardey Lukis was a sanitary commissioner with the Indian Government in 1911. Butler and Lukis were important figures in the research on malaria in India as members of the Indian Research Fund Association.
5. Stoler A.L. (2009) *Along the Archival Grain: Epistemic Anxieties and Colonial Common Sense*, Princeton: Princeton University Press, p. 95. Sara Ahmed uses the phrase 'moving' to describe the ways in which particular texts 'generate' particular 'effects'.
6. Ahmed S. (2004b) *The Cultural Politics of Emotion*, New York: Routledge.
7. Arnold D. (1992) *Colonizing the Body*, Berkeley: University of California Press. Arnold D. (1994) Public Health and Public Power: Medicine and Hegemony in Colonial India. In: Engels D. and Marks S. (eds) *Contesting Colonial Hegemony: State and Society in Africa and India* London: British Academic Press.
8. Harrison M. (1994) *Public Health in British India: Anglo-Indian Preventive Medicine, 1859–1914*, Cambridge: Cambridge University Press.
9. Wald P. (2008) *Contagious: Cultures, Carriers, and the Outbreak Narrative*, Durham, NC: Duke University Press.
10. Ibid., p. 26.
11. Metcalf T. (1998) *Ideologies of the Raj*, Cambridge: Cambridge University Press. Mehta U. (1997) *Liberal Strategies of Exclusion*, Berkeley: University of California Press.
12. Warwick Anderson labels these two as constituting the 'routines of colonial health work' in his article. Anderson W. (1998) Where Is the Postcolonial History of Medicine? *Bulletin of the History of Medicine* 72: 522–531.
13. Rosemary Fitzgerald uses this term in her essay. Fitzgerald R. (2001) *Clinical Christianity: The Emergence of Medical Work as a Missionary Strategy in Colonial India, 1800–1914*, Hyderabad: Orient Longman.
14. Bala P. (1991) *Imperialism and Medicine in Bengal: A Socio-Historical Perspective*, New Delhi: Sage Publications.

15. Ramasubban R. (1982) *Public Health and Medical Research in India: Their Origins under the Impact of British Colonial Policy*, Stockholm: SAREC.
16. Harrison, *Public Health in British India*.
17. Arnold Public Health and Public Power: Medicine and Hegemony in Colonial India.
18. Kumar A. (1998) *Medicine and the Raj: British Medical Policy in India, 1835–1911*, New Delhi: Sage Publications. Poovey M. (1988) *Uneven Developments: The Ideological Work of Gender in Mid-Victorian England*, Chicago: University of Chicago Press.
19. Poovey, *Uneven Developments*.
20. Arnold, *Colonizing the Body*. Ray K. (1998) *History of Public Health: Colonial Bengal, 1921–1947*, Calcutta: K.P. Bagchi and Company.
21. Kidambi P. (2007) *The Making of the Indian Metropolis*, New York: Ashgate.
22. Mushtaq M.U. (2009) Public Health in British India: A Brief Account of the History of Medical Services and Disease Prevention in Colonial India. *Indian Journal of Community Medicine* 34: 6–14.
23. Wald, *Contagious*, p. 26. Social contagion has been analyzed in several studies of affect and emotion in recent years. Gregg M. and Seigworth G.J. (2010) *The Affect Theory Reader*, Durham, NC: Duke University Press.
24. Ahmed S. (2010) Happy Objects. In: Gregg M. and Seigworth G.J. (eds) *The Affect Theory Reader*, Durham, NC: Duke University Press.
25. Pahari S. (1997) *Unish Satake Banglai Sanatani Chikitsha Byabastha* (Medical Systems in Nineteenth Century Bengal), Calcutta: Progressive Publishers.
26. Arnold D. and Sarkar S. (2001) In Search of Rational Remedies: Homoeopathy in Nineteenth Century Bengal. In: Ernst W. (ed.) *Plural Medicine, Tradition and Modernity, 1800–2000*, London: Routledge. Das S. (2011) Homoeopathic Families, Hindu Nation and the Legislating State: Making of a Vernacular Science, Bengal 1866–1941, PhD thesis, University College London.
27. Bala, *Imperialism and Medicine in Bengal*. Jeffery R. (1988) *The Politics of Health in India*, Berkeley: University of California Press.
28. Kumar A. (2001) *Indian Drug Industry under the Raj*, Hyderabad: Orient Longman.
29. Ackernecht E.H. (1973) *Therapeutics: From the Primitives to the 20th Century*, New York: Hafner Press.
30. Alter J.S. (2000b) *Gandhi's Body: Sex, Diet and the Politics of Nationalism*, Philadelphia: University of Pennsylvania Press.
31. Ramagundam R. (2008) *Gandhi's Khadi: A History of Contention and Conciliation*, Orient Blackswan Pvt. Ltd. Cohn B. (1996) Cloth, Clothes, and Colonialism: India in the Nineteenth Century. In: Cohn B. (ed.) *Colonialism and Its Forms of Knowledge*, Princeton, NJ: Princeton University Press, 106–162. Tarlo E. (1996) *Clothing Matters: Dress and Identity in India*, Chicago: University of Chicago Press. Gonsalves P. (2012) *Khadi: Gandhi's Mega Symbol of Subversion*, Thousand Oaks, CA: Sage Publications. Chakrabarty D. (1999) Clothing the Political Man: A Reading of the Use of Khadi/White in Indian Public Life. *Journal of Human Values*

5: 3–13. Bean S.S. (1989) Gandhi and Khadi: The Fabric of Independence. In: Scheider ABWaJ (ed.) *Cloth and Human Experience*, Washington, DC: Smithsonian Institution Press. Bayly C.A. (1999) *Empire and Information: Intelligence Gathering and Social Communication in India, 1780–1870*, Cambridge: Cambridge University Press.
32. Thrift N. (2010) Understanding the Material Practices of Glamour. In: Seigworth G.J. and Gregg M. (eds) *The Affect Theory Reader*, Durham, NC: Duke University Press. Turkle S. (2007a) *Evocative Objects: Things We Think With*, Boston: MIT Press.
33. Trift, Understanding the Material Practices of Glamour. Turkle, Evocative Objects.
34. Foucault M. (1982) *Archaeology of Knowledge*, New York: Vintage Books.
35. Lupton D. (1995) *The Imperative of Health: Public Health and the Regulated Body*, London: Sage.
36. Ahmed, *The Cultural Politics of Emotion*.
37. Walsh J. (2004) *Domesticity in Colonial India*, Lanham, MD: Rowman and Littlefield.
38. Veena Naregal elaborates how Anderson's thesis about print capitalism and the growth of modern vernacular cultures needs modification with respect to the colonial situation, where print entered as part of a modern capitalistic order but grew under circumstances inimical to the development of an indigenous market. Naregal V. (2001) *Language Politics, Elites, and the Public Sphere: Western India under Colonialism*, New Delhi: Permanent Black. Vernon J. (2007) *Hunger: A Modern History*, Cambridge, MA: Belknap Press. Also see Orsini F. (2002) *The Hindi Public Sphere, 1920–1940: Language and Literature in the Age of Nationalism*, Delhi: Oxford University Press.
39. Chatterjee P. (1995) *The Disciplines in Colonial Bengal*, Minneapolis: University of Minnesota Press.
40. Roy T. Disciplining the Printed Text: Colonial and Nationalist Surveillance of Bengali literature. In: Chatterjee. P. (ed.) *The Disciplines in Colonial Bengal*, Minneapolis: University of Minnesota Press.
41. Bose P.K. (1998) *Samayiki: Collection of Essays from Old Journals and Magazines: Volume One, Science and Society, 1850–1901*, Calcutta: Ananda Publishers.
42. Ibid., 1998: 16.
43. Chatterjee, *The Disciplines in Colonial Bengal*. Bayly, *Empire and Information*.
44. Basu A.R. (2004) Emergence of a marginal science in a colonial city: Reading psychiatry in Bengali periodicals. *The Indian Economic and Social History Review* 41: 103–141.
45. Berridge V. and Loughlin K. (2003) Glossary: Public Health History. *Journal of Epidemiology and Community Health* 57: 164–165. See also Petersen Alan and Lupton D. (1997b) *The New Public Health: Discourses, Knowledges, Strategies*, Thousand Oaks, CA: Sage Publications.
46. Gandhi M. (1949) *Diet and Diet Reform*, Ahmedabad: Navajivan Publishing House. Gandhi M. (1954) *Key to Health*, Ahmedabad: Navajivan Trust. Gandhi M. (1940c) *The Story of My Experiments with Truth*, Ahmedabad: Navajivan Press.

2 Alimentary Anxieties: Affect in Food and Hunger

1. What I mean by processes are the tropes of representations (that developed as part of the nationalist project), social and cultural imageries that defined and elucidated the actors, sites, practices, and kinds of bodies and processes that would build up the nation.
2. Farquhar J. and Hanson M.E. (1998) *Empires of Hygiene*, Durham, NC: Duke University Press.
3. Khare R.S. (1992) *The Eternal Food: Gastronomic Ideas and Influences of Hindus and Buddhists*, Albany, NY: Suny Press.
4. Appadurai A. (1981) Gastro-Politics in South Asia. *American Ethnologist* 3: 494–511.
5. Roy P. (2010) *Alimentary Tracts: Appetites, Aversions, and the Postcolonial*, Durham, NC: Duke University Press.
6. http://blogs.wsj.com/indiarealtime/2011/07/19/sketching-the-bengal-famine/. Accessed on January 2014. http://www.timeoutbengaluru.net/art/features/parched-art. Accessed on January 2014.
7. Mukherjee M. (2011) *Churchill's Dirty War: The British Empire and the Ravaging of India During World War II*, New York: Basic Books.
8. Hatty S. (1999) *The Disordered Body: Epidemic Disease and Cultural Transformation*, Albany, NY: Suny Press.
9. Campbell D. (2012) *The Iconography of Famine*, London: Reaktion Books.
10. Cooter R. (2010) *Visual Imagery and Epidemics in the Twentieth Century*, Minneapolis: University of Minnesota Press.
11. Jhabvala R.P. (1999) *Heat and Dust*, Berkeley: Counterpoint Press. Scott P. (1998) *The Jewel in the Crown. (The Raj Quartet)*, Chicago: University of Chicago Press.
12. Ray K. (1998) *History of Public Health: Colonial Bengal, 1921–1947*, Calcutta: K.P. Bagchi and Company.
13. Ibid., p. 255.
14. Ibid.
15. Hardgrove A. (2005) *Community and Public Culture: The Marwaris in Calcutta 1897–1997*, New York: Columbia University Press (Gutenberg E.).
16. Prasad S. (2006) Crisis, Identity, and Social Distinction: Cultural Politics of Food, Taste, and Consumption in Late Colonial Bengal. *Journal of Historical Sociology* 19(3): 246–265.
17. Fisher J. Tea and Food Adulteration, 1834–75. In: Felluga D.F. (ed.) *BRANCH Britain, Representation and Nineteenth-Century History*. http://www.branchcollective.org/?ps_articles=judith-l-fisher-tea-and-food-adulteration-1834-75.
18. Bayly C.A. (1992) *The Origins of Swadeshi: Cloth and Indian Society, 1700–1930*, Cambridge: Cambridge University Press.
19. Prasad, Crisis, Identity, and Social Distinction.
20. Guha S. (1925) *Swasthya Samashya*, Calcutta.
21. Bhattacharya N.C. (1935) *Bangalir Khadya O Pushti* (The Health and Nutrition of Bengalis), Calcutta.
22. Ray P.C. (1936) *Anna Samasyay Bangalir Parajoy o Tahar Pratikar* (The Food Crisis, Bengali's Defeat and its Remedy), Calcutta: Ranjan Publishing

House. Das S.M. (1935) *Basu, Chunilal*, Calcutta: Khadya. Sen K.I. (1928) *Bangalir Khadya* (A Handbook on the Principles of Bengali Dietetics), Calcutta: ArogyaNiketan. Ray U. (2012) Constructing a 'Pure' Body: The Discourse of Nutrition in Colonial Bengal. Institute of Development Studies Occasional Paper 40.
23. Ibid., p. 11.
24. Ibid., p. 15.
25. Ahmed S. (2004a) *Affective Economies*, Social Text 22.
26. http://www.open.edu/openlearn/history-the-arts/history/social-econo mic-history/listen-the-bengal-famine. Accessed on 6 March 2014.
27. http://blogs.wsj.com/indiarealtime/2011/07/19/sketching-the-bengal-famine/; http://www.delhiartgallery.com/exhibition/exhibition.aspx?ExId=56&city=DLI accessed on 7 March 2014. Somnath Hore's collection of lithographs, ink sketches, and drawings on the Bengal Famine of 1943 was exhibited in December 2013; and Chatterjee M. A look at Bengal Famine in Modern Indian Art – a Showcase Leads the Way, My Blog: A Fine Wordpress.com site. https://madhusreechatterjee.wordpress.com/2013/12/26/a-look-at-bengal-famine-in-modern-indian-art-a-showcase-leads-the-way/.
28. McLean S. (2004) *The Event and Its Terrors: Ireland, Famine, and Modernity*, Stanford: Stanford University Press.
29. Arnold D. (1988) *Famine: Social Crisis and Historical Change*, Oxford: Basil Blackwell.
30. Morash C. (1995) *Writing the Irish Famine*, Oxford: Clarendon Press.
31. Greenough P. (1982) *Prosperity and Misery in Modern Bengal: The Famine of 1943–1944*, New York: Oxford University Press.
32. Ibid., pp. vii–viii.
33. Kelleher M. (1997) *The Feminization of Famine: Expressions of the Inexpressible?* Durham: Duke University Press.
34. Weisenfeld G. (2012) *Imaging Disaster: Tokyo and the Visual Culture of Japan's Great Earthquake of 1923*, Berkeley: University of California Press.
35. Morash, *Writing the Irish Famine*. McLean, *The Event and Its Terrors*.
36. http://www.thedelhiwalla.com/2011/07/18/city-culture-chittaprosads-retrospective-delhi-art-gallery/. Accessed on 18 April 2014.
37. Eaton N. (2013) *Colour, Art and Empire: Visual Culture and the Nomadism of Representation*, London: I.B. Tauris.
38. Dasgupta R. (2014) 'The People' in People's Art and People's War. In: Chakarabarty G. (ed.) *People's Warrior: Words and Worlds of P.C. Joshi*. Calcutta: Tulika, 443–456.
39. Ibid., p. 451.
40. Ibid., p. 452.
41. Ibid., p. 450.
42. Vernon J. (2007) *Hunger: A Modern History*, Cambridge, MA: Belknap Press.

3 Body, Hygiene, and the Affective Politics of Gandhi's *Swaraj*

1. Alter J. (2000a) *Gandhi's Body: Sex, Diet, and the Politics of Nationalism*, Philadelphia: University of Pennsylvania Press.

2. I have borrowed the term 'biomoral' from Joseph Alter's seminal work on the centrality of the body to Gandhian thought and politics.
3. I have borrowed my use of the term 'experiment' from Tridip Suhrud's essay on Gandhi's seminal writings. He comments on why Gandhi chose the term '*prayogo*' or experiment over '*sadhana*' or spiritual practice. For a discussion on this see Suhrud T. (2011) *Gandhi's Key Writings: In Search of Unity*, Cambridge: Cambridge University Press.
4. Birla R. and Devji F. (2011) Guest Editor's Letter: Itineraries of Self-Rule. *Public Culture* 23: 265–268. Arjun Appadurai writes how he feels that Gandhi is the 'right figure to stimulate this engagement, for he had a famous disregard for history as fact, chronology, or destiny. Yet he is himself utterly unthinkable apart from his special history, which took him from Gujarat to England, from England to South Africa, and from South Africa back to India'. See Appadurai A. (2011) Our Gandhi, Our Times. *Public Culture* 23(2).
5. Birla, Guest Editor's Letter, p. 265.
6. Alter J.S. (2000b) Gandhi's Body: Sex, Diet and the Politics of Nationalism Philadelphia: University of Pennsylvania Press, p. xv.
7. Amit Misra makes a similar point in his essay, (2001) 'Public Health Issues and the Freedom Movement: Gandhi on Nutrition, Sanitation, and Infectious Diseases and Health Care, In: Kumar D. (ed.), *Disease and Medicine in India: A Historical Overview* New Delhi, India. Tulika Books. See also Misra A. (2004) *Public Health Issues and the Freedom Movement: Gandhi on Nutrition, Sanitation, and Infectious Diseases and Health Care*, New Delhi: Manohar.
8. Gandhi M. (1940b) *Sanitary Reform and Famine Relief*, Ahmedabad: Navjivan Press.
9. Ibid.
10. Alter, (2000b) *Gandhi's Body*, p. 7.
11. Sarkar T. (2011) *Gandhi and Social Relations*, Cambridge: Cambridge University Press.
12. Ibid., p. 190.
13. Skaria A. (2010) Living by Dying. In: Anand Pandian and Daud Ali (eds) *In Ethical Life in South Asia*, Bloomington: Indiana University Press.
14. Gandhi M. (1933) *Self-Restraint versus Self-Indulgence*, Ahmedabad: Navajivan Press.
15. Gandhi, *The Story of My Experiments with Truth*.
16. Ibid., p. 406.
17. Alter, *Gandhi's Body*. Also see Bala S. (2008) The Dramaturgy of Fasting in Gandhian Nonviolent Action. In: Wagner Meike and Ernst W.D. (eds) *Performing the Matrix: Mediating Cultural Performances*. München: ePODIUM, pp. 289–306.
18. Gandhi M. (1940a) *Fasting as Penance*, Ahmedabad: Navajivan Press.
19. Hofmeyr I. (2013) *Fasting as Penance*, Cambridge: Harvard University Press.
20. Gandhi M. (1899) The Plague Panic in South Africa. This article was originally published in the *Times of India* in April 1899.

21. Burton A. (2012) *Brown over Black: Race and the Politics of Postcolonial Citation*, Gurgaon: Three Essays Collective. See also another piece by Gandhi where he voices the concern that the physician who is treating a patient might sometimes need a treatment himself. He criticizes the Durban Town Council for unjustly and forcefully segregating Indians in that area and therefore needing some reflection on their part. See Gandhi M. (1903) Physician Heal Thyself. This piece was originally published in *Indian Opinion* in June 1903.
22. Gandhi M. (1904c) The Plague in the Transvaal. This article was originally published in *Indian Opinion* in April 1904. Gandhi M. (1904b) The Plague. This article was also originally published in *Indian Opinion* in April 1904.
23. Gandhi M. (1904a) A Lesson from the Plague. This piece was originally published in *Indian Opinion* in April 1904.
24. Gandhi M. (1904d) The Plague Peg. This was originally published in *Indian Opinion* in July 1904. See also Gandhi, (1904b) The Plague, p. 331. This article was originally published in *Indian Opinion* in January 1905. Sarkar, *Gandhi and Social Relations*.
25. There is a rich body of scholarship that has analyzed the transnational linkages of Gandhi's nationalist politics. Among them is Hofmeyr (2013) *Gandhi's Printing Press*.
26. Gandhi M. (1905a) Malaria in Durban. This piece was originally published in April 1905 in *Indian Opinion*. Gandhi M. (1905b) Smallpox in Johannesburg. This was written in May 1905 for *Indian Opinion*.
27. Gandhi M. (1910) *Hind Swaraj*. p. 53.
28. Ibid. Misra (2004) *Public Health Issues and the Freedom Movement*.
29. Sandhya Shetty rightly points out, 'No other thinker from within the ranks of decolonization has presented as robust and radical a critique of medicine as has Mohandas Karamchand Gandhi'. See Shetty S. (2008) *The Quack Whom We Know: Illness and Nursing in Gandhi*, London: Routledge. Ibid. p. 38.
30. Gandhi, M. CW (Collective Works of Mahatma Gandhi), Volume 11, 1911–1913, pp. 434, 441, 447, 453, 458, 463, 467, 472, and 479. See also CW Volume 12, pp. 4, 62. Most of these articles were first published in the *Indian Opinion*.

4 Imagining the Social Body: Competing Moralities of Care and Contagion

1. Forbes G. (1994) Medical Careers and Health Care for Indian Women: patterns of control. *Women's History Review* 3: 515–530. Lal M. (1994) The Politics of Gender and Medicine in Colonial India: The Countess of Dufferin's Fund, 1885–1888. *Bulletin for History of Medicine* 68: 29–66.
2. Karlekar M. (1986) Kadambini and the Bhadralok: Early Debates over Women's Education in Bengal. *Economic and Political Weekly* XXI: 25–31. Deb C. (1998) *Mahila Daktar: Bhin Graher Bashinda*, Calcutta: Ananda Publishers.

3. Forbes G. and Raychaudhuri T. (2000) *Memoirs of Haimabati Sen: From Child Widow to Lady Doctor*, New Delhi: Roli Books.
4. Borthwick M. (1984) *The Changing Role of Women in Bengal 1849–1905*, Princeton: Princeton University Press.
5. Ibid.
6. Mukherjee M. (1995) *Women's Work in Bengal, 1880–1930: A Historical Analysis*, Delhi: Oxford University Press.
7. Forbes G. (2000a) *Women in Modern India*, Cambridge: Cambridge University Press.
8. Office of the Superintendent. (1908) *Twenty-Third Annual Report of the National Association for Supplying Female Medical Aid to the Women of India*. Calcutta: Office of the Superintendent, pp. 10–12.
9. Ibid.
10. Balfour M.I. and Young R. (1929) *The Work of Medical Women in India*, London: Oxford University Press.
11. Desivilliar R.C. (1920) Child Welfare and Infant Mortality. *Journal of Association of Medical Women in India* 3: 5–11. Desivilliar was the editor of the Local Self Government Gazette.
12. Mukherjee S. (2001) *Disciplining the Body? Health Care for Women and Children in Early Twentieth Century Bengal*, New Delhi: Tulika.
13. Ray B. (2001) *Women, Politics and Identity in Colonial Bengal, 1900–1947*, Calcutta: K.P. Bagchi and Company.
14. Basu A. and Ray B. (1990) *Women's Struggle: A History of the All India Women's Conference 1927–1990*, Delhi: Manohar Books.
15. Editor of *Rachanasamgraha*: Shukhalata Rao states that it is not known when *Pather Alo* was written, but that it was certainly after 1937. See Appendix, Shukhalata Rao: *Rachanasamgraha* Volume I (1999) Calcutta: Thema, p. 229.
16. Sarkar T. (1999) *Words to Win: The Making of Amar Jiban: A Modern Autobiography*, New Delhi: Kali for Women.
17. Ibid., p. 3. There are a number of autobiographies and memoirs by Indian women writers for whom becoming literate and educated, and being able to write were turning points in their lives. See Forbes G. and Raychaudhuri T. (2000b) *The Memoirs of Dr Haimabati Sen: From Child Widow to Lady Doctor*, New Delhi: Roli Books. Bandyopadhyay A.K. and Sen A. (1998) *Purnashashi Debir-r Nirbachita Rachana* (Selected Writings of Purnashashi Debi), Calcutta: Deys Publishing. See also Gupta R. (1999b) *Smritimanjusha: Priyabala Gupta*, Calcutta.
There were women from elite and well-known families who faced no apparent restrictions as far as their education was concerned and went on to become active and prominent literary, social reform, or political figures. Forbes G. (2005) *Women in Colonial India: Essays on Politics, Medicine and Historiography*, San Francisco: Chronicle Books. Burton A. (1996) Contesting the Zenana: The Mission to Make 'Lady Doctors for India, 1874–1885'. *Journal of British Studies* 35: 368–397. Karlekar (1986) *Economic and Political Weekly* XXI: 25–31.

18. I use the term 'new knowledge' from Sidonie Smith and Julia Watson's essay where they discuss how 'agency' becomes central to discussions of women's autobiographies. See Smith S. (1998) *Women, Autobiography, Theory: A Reader*, Madison: University of Wisconsin Press.
19. Rao S. (19–) *Pather Alo*, Calcutta, pp. 67–68.
20. Gupta R. (1999a) *Alor Abhimukhe: The Life and Times of Priyabala Gupta*, Calcutta: Dey's Publishers, p. 133.
21. Debi P. (1941) *Smritimanjusha*, Calcutta: Dey's Publishers.
22. Bandyopadhyay A. (1998) *The Way I Have Seen Purnashashi*, Calcutta: Dey's Publishers, p. 27.
23. Gigliotti S. (2002) *Technology, Trauma and Representation: Holocaust Testimony and Videotape*, Manchester: Manchester University Press.
24. *Pather Alo*, p. 71.
25. Ibid., pp. 71–72.
26. Dyson L. (2002) *Collecting Practices and Autobiography: The Role of Objects in the Mnemonic Landscape of Nation*, Manchester: Manchester University Press, p. 129.
27. Ibid.
28. Ibid.
29. Turkle S. (2007b) *What Makes an Object Evocative?* Cambridge, MA: MIT Press, p. 307.
30. Petersen A. (1997a) *The New Public Health: Discourses, Knowledge, Strategies*, Thousand Oaks, CA: Sage Publications.
31. Bagchi J. (1999) Preface, 'The Light of Your Life'. In: Gupta R. (ed.) *Smritimanjusha*. Calcutta: Dey's Publishing.
32. Ibid.
33. Gupta P. (1963) *Smritimanjusha*, p. 46.
34. Ibid., p. 59.
35. Bagchi, Preface, 'The light of your life'.
36. Ibid., pp. 10–13.
37. Ibid., p. 46.
38. Ibid., p. 59.
39. Ibid., p. 63.
40. Sarkar, *Words to Win*, p. 8.
41. Ibid., p. 71.
42. Ibid., p. 91.
43. Smith (1998) *Women, Autobiography, Theory*.
44. Much has been written on the discourse that was at its peak around 1900 about the horrific realities of the *zenana* – an archaic, primitive space which stifled women's lives. Many of Priyabala Gupta's representations of house and home exude the same kind of negativity with which the term *zenana* was associated. See Burton A. (2003) *Dwelling in the Archives: Women Writing House, Home, and History in Late Colonial India*, Oxford: Oxford University Press, p. 11.
45. Ibid., p. 15.
46. Deb (1998) *Mahila Daktar*.
47. Debi P. (1963) *Mone Pare*, Calcutta, p. 223.

48. Ibid., p. 229.
49. Ibid., p. 219.
50. Ibid.
51. Ibid., p. 225.
52. Ibid., p. 247.
53. Ibid., p. 257.
54. Deb, *Mahila Daktar*, p. 13.
55. Ibid., p. 353.
56. Ibid. Sarkar, *Words to Win*.

5 Affective Remedies: Advertisements and Cultural Politics of Hygiene

1. Ciarlo D. (2011) *Advertising Empire: Race and Visual Culture in Imperial Germany*, Cambridge: Harvard University Press, p. 4.
2. See Landy J. and Saler M. (2009) *The Re-Enchantment of the World: Secular Magic in a Rational Age*, Stanford: Stanford University Press. Also see https://www.ned.univie.ac.at/sites/default/files/20505/saler%202.pdf.
3. Ibid., p. 2.
4. Saler M. (2006) Modernity and Enchantment: A Historiographic Review. *American Historical Review* 111 (3): 692–716.
5. Ibid., p. 692.
6. Dube S. (2009) *Enchantments of Modernity: Empire, Nation, and Globalization*, London: Routledge.
7. Ibid., p. 1.
8. Ibid., p. 30.
9. Ibid., p. 5.
10. Bennett J. (2001) *The Enchantment of Modernity: Attachments, Crossings, and Ethics*, Princeton: Princeton University Press.
11. Ibid., p. 8.
12. Ibid., p. 114.
13. Jay M. and Ramaswamy S.R. (2014) *Empires of Vision: A Reader*, Durham: Duke University Press.
14. Richards T. (1990) *The Commodity Culture of Victorian England*, Stanford: Stanford University Press, p. 54.
15. Ibid., p. 55.
16. McClintock A. (1995) *Imperial Leather: Race, Gender and Sexuality in the Colonial Contest*, New York: Routledge, p. 211.
17. Burke T. (1996) *Lifebuoy Men, Lux Women: Commodification, Consumption, and Cleanliness in Modern Zimbabwe*, Durham: Duke University Press.
18. See in this context *Medical Fringe and Medical Orthodoxy, 1750–1850*, edited by W.F. Bynum and Roy Porter who challenge the supposed enmity and outright war between patent medicine and rational-scientific medicine; Bynum W.F. (1987) *Medical Fringe and Medical Orthodoxy, 1750–1850*, London: Croom Helm. The book maps the relationship between 'regular' and 'irregular' medicines in the particular historical contexts

of Europe and America. In the past 15 years, the terms of the debate have changed and the validity of narrow dualisms such as orthodoxy versus fringe or mainstream versus alternative/subaltern has been increasingly questioned. For example, the essays in *Plural Medicine, Tradition and Modernity, 1800–2000*, which belong to this new genre of research, consider it imperative to look into parallel histories of medicine and their interaction in a much more 'plural' and yet power-laden field. Ernst W. (2002) *Plural Medicine, Tradition and Modernity, 1800–2000*, London: Routledge, p. 253.
19. Kumar A. (2001) *Indian Drug Industry under the Raj*, Hyderabad: Orient Longman.
20. Pahari S. (1997) *Unish Satake Banglai Sanatani Chikitsha Byabastha* (Medical Systems in Nineteenth Century Bengal), Calcutta: Progressive Publishers.
21. Arnold D. and Sarkar S. (2001) In Search of Rational Remedies: Homoeopathy in Nineteenth Century Bengal. In: Ernst W. (ed.) *Plural Medicine, Tradition and Modernity, 1800*–2000, London: Routledge. See also Roy B. (1995a) *Unish Satake Deshiya Bhashai Chikitshabigyan Charcha* (The Pursuit of Medical Science in the Nineteenth Century in the Vernacular), Kolkata: Ananda Publishers.
22. There is a body of scholarship on medical history in the context of India, which has explored the rich history of the development, consolidation, and shifts in local medical traditions like *unani*, *hakimi*, homeopathic, and Ayurvedic methods in the nineteenth and early twentieth centuries; See for example, Attewell G. (2007) *Refiguring Unani Tibb: Plural Healing in Late Colonial India*, Hyderabad: Orient Longman. Das S. (2011) *Homoeopathic Families, Hindu Nation and the Legislating State: Making of a Vernacular Science, Bengal 1866–1941*, London: University College London. Liebeskind C. (2014) Arguing Science: Unani Tibb, Hakims, and Biomedicine in India, 1900–1950. In: Ernst W. (ed.) *Plural Medicine, Tradition and Modernity, 1800–2000*. London: Routledge. Kumar D. (1997) Unequal Contenders, Uneven Ground: Medical Encounters in British India, 1820–1920. In: Andrews B. and Sutphen M. P. (eds) *Western Medicine as Contested Knowledge*, London: Routledge.
23. Anonymous. (1886) *Chikitsa Sammilani*.
24. Mishra D. (1987) *Advertising in Indian Newspapers, 1780–1947*, Behrampur: Ishani Publications.
25. Kumar A. (1998) *Medicine and the Raj: British Medical Policy in India, 1835–1911*, New Delhi: Sage Publications.
26. The *Indian Mirror* was started in 1861 with Keshabchandra Sen, the Brahmo reformer, as the editor.
27. The *Indian Mirror*, 1889. See also Sharma M. (2009) Creating a Consumer: Exploring Medical Advertisements in Colonial India. In: Harrison M. and Pati B. (eds) *The Social History of Health and Medicine in Colonial India*, London: Routledge.
28. http://www.pitara.com/discover/5wh/104.htm.
29. *Amrita Bazar Patrika*, 1905.

30. Sharma, Creating a Consumer, p. 219.
31. *The Hindoo Patriot* was a weekly English newspaper, first published in January 1853 under the proprietorship of Madhusudhan Roy with Girish Chandra Ghosh as the Managing Editor. Under the ownership of Harishchandra Mukherjee, *The Hindoo Patriot* played a vital role in bringing to light the tyranny of Indigo planters, in the post-Mutiny period. Regular editorials against such tyranny on the poor hapless indigo raiyats attracted public attention and evoked universal condemnation from a large cross-section of educated Indians. Other principal social issues highlighted by the Patriot in its columns were female education and Hindu widow remarriage. As regards female education, the paper advised everybody to follow the lead given by John Drinkwater Bethune and on the question of widow remarriage it sided with the reformists and supported the cause of legalizing such marriages. The paper, however, opposed the implementation of divorce laws in Hindu society. Although the principal objective of *The Hindoo Patriot* was to shed light upon negative aspects of the anomalies in British Government in India, it pinned very high hopes on the liberalism of the British public and parliament. Thus, it always advised Indians to address their grievances to the British public and parliament whenever the British Indian administration failed to redress their complaints. The focus on the negative aspects of British rule was not intended to tarnish the image of the British Indian government.
32. *Amrita Bazar Patrika*, 1923.
33. *The Bengalee*, 1932, p. 3.
34. *The Statesman*, 1925.
35. http://www.magindia.com/history.hist2.html.
36. *Chikitsa Sammilani*, 1897.
37. http://www.cssscal.org/.
38. *Grihasthamangal*, 1931.
39. Ibid.
40. Burke, *Lifebuoy Men, Lux Women*.
41. *Grihasthamangal*, 1928, Number 6.
42. It is interesting in this context to note analysis of pictorial techniques used in American advertisements. These pictorial representations commonly followed what Jackson Lears describes for advertising in America

   > Breath and body perfumes, talcum powder and toilet water, all were placed in settings redolent with luxurious sensuality. There was a strikingly overt eroticism about many of these images, in specific icons and more generally in the air of the languorous ease displayed by the mature and voluptuous women, whom historians of fashion have identified as the beau ideal of the late 19th century.
   >
   > (Lears J. [1994] *Fables of Abundance: A Cultural History of Advertising in America*, New York: Basic Books)

43. *The Statesman*.
44. Ibid.

45. According to Raymond Williams, patent food was one of the most heavily advertised products in the late nineteenth century besides new inventions like the sewing machine, the camera, the bicycle and the typewriter. See Williams R. (1993) Advertising: The Magic System. In: During S. (ed.) *The Cultural Studies Reader*, London: Routledge.
46. Lears, *Fables of Abundance*. Anne McClintock alludes to something of a similar phenomenon, where commodities become the epitomes of civilization itself. She characterizes much of imperial advertising as marking a strong degree of 'commodity racism' and an 'imperial spectacle', which draws stark and unbridgeable contrasts between the civilized empire and the savage colonies; See McClintock (1995) *Imperial Leather*.
47. The *Statesman*, The Bengalee, and Advance.
48. Goldman R. (1992) *Reading Ads Socially*, London: Routledge.
49. Festa L. (2006) *Sentimental Figure of Empire in Eighteenth-Century Britain and France*, Baltimore: Johns Hopkins Press, p. 6.
50. Ibid., p. 3.
51. Ahmed S. (2004b) *The Cultural Politics of Emotion*, New York: Routledge, p. 12.
52. Ibid.
53. Stage S. and Vincenti B.V. (1997) *Rethinking Home Economics: Women and the History of a Profession*, Ithaca: Cornell University Press. Tomes N. (1998) *The Gospel of Germs: Men, Women, and the Microbe in American Life*, Cambridge, MA: Harvard University Press.

Conclusion

1. Chakrabarty H. (1894) *Olautha Nibaraner Upai*, Calcutta: *Chikitsa Sammilani*. p. 92.
2. Ibid.
3. Epstein H. (2014) *Ebola in Liberia: An Epidemic of Rumors*. New York: The New York Review of Books LXI.
4. Bashford A. and Hooker C. (2001) *Contagion*, London: Routledge.

References

Ackerknecht E.H. (1973) *Therapeutics: From the Primitives to the 20th Century*, New York: Hafner Press.
Ahmed S. (2004a) Affective Economies. *Social Text* 22 (2): 117–139.
Ahmed S. (2004b) *The Cultural Politics of Emotion*, New York: Routledge.
Ahmed S. (2010) Happy Objects. In: Gregg M. and Seigworth G.J. (eds) *The Affect Theory Reader*, Duke: Duke University Press.
Alter J. (2000a) *Gandhi's Body: Sex, Diet, and the Politics of Nationalism*, Philadelphia: University of Pennsylvania Press.
Alter J.S. (2000b) *Gandhi's Body: Sex, Diet and the Politics of Nationalism*, Philadelphia: University of Pennsylvania Press.
Anderson W. (1998) Where Is the Postcolonial History of Medicine? *Bulletin of the History of Medicine* 72: 522–531.
Anonymous (1886) *Chikitsa Sammilani*.
Appadurai A. (1981) Gastro-Politics in South Asia. *American Ethnologist* 3: 494–511.
Appadurai A. (2011) Our Gandhi, Our Times. *Public Culture* 23 (2): 263–264.
Arnold D. (1988) *Famine: Social Crisis and Historical Change*, Oxford: Basil Blackwell.
Arnold D. (1992) *Colonizing the Body*, Berkeley: University of California Press.
Arnold D. (1994) Public Health and Public Power: Medicine and Hegemony in Colonial India. In: Engels D. and Marks S. (eds) *Contesting Colonial Hegemony: State and Society in Africa and India*, London: British Academic Press.
Arnold D. and Sarkar S. (2001) In Search of Rational Remedies: Homoeopathy in Nineteenth Century Bengal. In: Ernst W. (ed.) *Plural Medicine, Tradition and Modernity, 1800–2000*, London: Routledge.
Attewell G. (2007) *Refiguring Unani Tibb: Plural Healing in Late Colonial India*, Hyderabad: Orient Longman.
Bagchi J. (1999) Preface, 'The Light of Your Life'. In: Gupta R. (ed.) *Smritimanjusha*, Kolkata: Dey's Publishers.
Bala P. (1991) *Imperialism and Medicine in Bengal: A Socio-Historical Perspective*, New Delhi: Sage Publications.
Bala S. (2008) The Dramaturgy of Fasting in Gandhian Nonviolent Action. In: Wagner Meike and Ernst W.D. (eds) *Performing the Matrix: Mediating Cultural Performances*, München: ePODIUM, pp. 289–306.
Balfour M.I. and Young R. (1929) *The Work of Medical Women in India*, London: Oxford University Press.
Bandyopadhyay A. (1998) *The Way I Have Seen Purnashashi*, Kolkata: Dey's Publishers.

Bandyopadhyay A.K. and Sen A. (1998) *Purnashashi Debir-r Nirbachita Rachana (Selected Writings of Purnashashi Debi)*, Kolkata: Dey's Publishers.
Bashford A. and Hooker C. (2001) *Contagion*, London: Routledge.
Basu A. and Ray B. (1990) *Women's Struggle: A History of the All India Women's Conference 1927–1990*, Delhi: Manohar Books.
Basu A.R. (2004) Emergence of a Marginal Science in a Colonial City: Reading Psychiatry in Bengali Periodicals. *The Indian Economic and Social History Review* 41: 103–141.
Bayly C.A. (1992) *The Origins of Swadeshi: Cloth and Indian Society, 1700–1930*, Cambridge: Cambridge University Press.
Bayly C.A. (1999) *Empire and Information: Intelligence Gathering and Social Communication in India, 1780–1870*, Cambridge: Cambridge University Press.
Bean S.S. (1989) Gandi and Khadi: The Fabric of Independence. In: Weiner A. and Schneider J. (eds) *Cloth and Human Experience*, Washington, DC: Smithsonian Institution Press.
Bennett J. (2001) *The Enchantment of Modernity: Attachments, Crossings, and Ethics*, Princeton: Princeton University Press.
Berridge V. and Loughlin K. (2003) Glossary: Public Health History. *Journal of Epidemiology and Community Health* 57: 164–165.
Bhattacharya N.C. (1935) *Bangalir Khadya O Pushti (The Health and Nutrition of Bengalis)*, Kolkata.
Birla R. and Devji F. (2011) Guest Editor's Letter: Itineraries of Self-Rule. *Public Culture* 23: 265–268.
Borthwick M. (1984) *The Changing Role of Women in Bengal 1849–1905*, Princeton: Princeton University Press.
Bose P.K. (1998) *Samayiki: Collection of Essays from Old Journals and Magazines: Volume One, Science and Society, 1850–1901*, Calcutta: Ananda Publishers.
Burke T. (1996) *Lifebuoy Men, Lux Women: Commodification, Consumption, and Cleanliness in Modern Zimbabwe*, Durham: Duke University Press.
Burton A. (1996) Contesting the Zenana: The Mission to Make 'Lady Doctors for India, 1874–1885', *Journal of British Studies* 35: 368–397.
Burton A. (2003) *Dwelling in the Archives: Women Writing House, Home, and History in Late Colonial India*, Oxford: Oxford University Press.
Burton A. (2012) *Brown over Black: Race and the Politics of Postcolonial Citation*, Gurgaon: Three Essays Collective.
Butler, Spencer Harcourt. (1912) The Second All-India Sanitary Conference Opening Speech. In: *The Proceedings of the Second All-India Sanitary Conference*. Madras.
Bynum W.F. and Porter R. (1987) *Medical Fringe and Medical Orthodoxy, 1750–1850*, London: Croom Helm.
Campbell D. (2012) *The Iconography of Famine*, London: Reaktion Books.
Chakrabarty D. (1999) Clothing the Political Man: A Reading of the Use of Khadi/White in Indian Public Life. *Journal of Human Values* 5: 3–13.
Chakrabarty H. (1894) *Olautha Nibaraner Upai*. Chikitsa Sammilani. Calcutta: Sharat Shashi Jantra, Calcutta

Chatterjee M. (26 December 2013) A *Look at Bengal Famine in Modern Indian Art – a Showcase Leads the Way*, My Blog: A Fine Wordpress.com site. https://madhusreechatterjee.wordpress.com/2013/12/26/a-look-at-bengal-famine-in-modern-indian-art-a-showcase-leads-the-way/.

Chatterjee P (ed.). (1995) *The Disciplines in Colonial Bengal*, Minneapolis: University of Minnesota Press.

Ciarlo D. (2011) *Advertising Empire: Race and Visual Culture in Imperial Germany*, Cambridge: Harvard University Press.

Cohn B. (1996) *Cloth, Clothes, and Colonialism: India in the Nineteenth Century. Colonialism and Its Forms of Knowledge*, Princeton, NJ: Princeton University Press.

Cooter R. (2010) *Visual Imagery and Epidemics in the Twentieth Century*, Minneapolis: University of Minnesota Press.

Das S. (2011) *Homoeopathic Families, Hindu Nation and the Legislating State: Making of a Vernacular Science, Bengal 1866–1941*, London: University College London.

Das S.M. (1935) *Basu, Chunilal*, Kolkata: Khadya.

Dasgupta R. (2014) The People in People's Art and People's War. In: Chakarabarty G. (ed.) *People's Warrior: Words and Worlds of P.C. Joshi*. Kolkata: Tulika, pp. 443–456.

Deb C. (1998) *Mahila Daktar: Bhin Graher Bashinda*, Kolkata: Ananda Publishers.

Debi P. (1941) *Smritimanjusha*, Kolkata: Dey's Publishers.

Debi P. (1963) *Mone Pare*, Kolkata: Dey's Publishing, Calcutta

Desivilliar R.C. (1920) Child Welfare and Infant Mortality. *Journal of Association of Medical Women in India* 3: 5–11.

Dube S. (2009) *Enchantments of Modernity: Empire, Nation, and Globalization*, New Delhi: Routledge.

Dyson L. (2002) *Collecting Practices and Autobiography: The Role of Objects in the Mnemonic Landscape of Nation*, Manchester: Manchester University Press.

Eaton N. (2013) *Colour, Art and Empire: Visual Culture and the Nomadism of Representation*, London: I.B. Tauris.

Epstein H. (2014) *Ebola in Liberia: An Epidemic of Rumors*, New York: The New York Review of Books LXI.

Ernst W. (2002) *Plural Medicine, Tradition and Modernity, 1800–2000*, London: Routledge. p. 253.

Farquhar J. and Hanson M. (1998) *Empires of Hygiene*, Durham: Duke University Press.

Festa L. (2006) *Sentimental Figure of Empire in Eighteenth-Century Britain and France*, Baltimore: Johns Hopkins Press.

Fisher J. Tea and Food Adulteration, 1834–75. In: Felluga D.F. (ed.) *BRANCH Britain, Representation and Nineteenth-Century History*.

Fitzgerald R. (2001) *Clinical Christianity: The Emergence of Medical Work as a Missionary Strategy in Colonial India, 1800–1914*, Hyderabad: Orient Longman.

Forbes G. (1994) Medical Careers and Health Care for Indian Women: Patterns of Control. *Women's History Review* 3: 515–530.
Forbes G. (2000a) *Women in Modern India*, Cambridge: Cambridge University Press.
Forbes G. and Raychaudhuri T. (2000b) *The Memoirs of Dr Haimabati Sen: From Child Widow to Lady Doctor*, New Delhi: Roli Books.
Forbes G. (2005) *Women in Colonial India: Essays on Politics, Medicine and Historiography*, New Delhi: Chronicle Books.
Foucault M. (1982) *Archaeology of Knowledge*, New York: Vintage Books.
Gandhi M. (1899) The Plague Panic in South Africa (*The Times of India*, 22-4-1899).
Gandhi M. (1903) Physician Heal Thyself (Indian Opinion, 18-6-1903).
Gandhi M. (1904a) A Lesson From The Plague (Indian Opinion, 30-4-1904).
Gandhi M. (1904b) The Plague (Indian Opinion, 23-4-1904).
Gandhi M. (1904c) The Plague in the Transvaal (Indian Opinion, 9-4-1904).
Gandhi M. (1904d) The Plague Peg (Indian Opinion, 16-7-1904).
Gandhi M. (1905a) Malaria in Durban (Indian Opinion, 22-4-1905).
Gandhi M. (1905b) Smallpox Epidemic in Johannesburg (Indian Opinion, 3-6-1905).
Gandhi M. (1910) *Hind Swaraj*, p. 53.
Gandhi M. (1933) *Self-Restraint versus Self-Indulgence*, Ahmedabad: Navajivan Publishing House.
Gandhi M. (1940a) *Fasting as Penance*, Ahmedabad: Navajivan Press.
Gandhi M. (1940b) *Sanitary Reform and Famine Relief*, Ahmedabad: Navjivan Press.
Gandhi M. (1940c) *The Story of My Experiments with Truth*, Ahmedabad: Navajivan Press.
Gandhi M. (1949) *Diet and Diet Reform*, Ahmedabad: Navajivan Publishing House.
Gandhi M. (1954) *Key to Health*, Ahmedabad: Navajivan Publishing House.
Gigliotti S. (2002) *Technology, Trauma and Representation: Holocaust Testimony and Videotape*, Manchester: Manchester University Press.
Goldman R. (1992) *Reading Ads Socially*, London: Routledge.
Gonsalves P. (2012) *Khadi: Gandhi's Mega Symbol of Subversion*, New Delhi: Sage Publications.
Greenough P. (1982) *Prosperity and Misery in Modern Bengal: The Famine of 1943–1944*, New York: Oxford University Press.
Gregg M. and Seigworth G.J. (2010) *The Affect Theory Reader*, Durham: Duke University Press.
Guha S. (1925) *Swasthya Samashya*, Calcutta.
Gupta P. (1963) *Smritimanjusha*. Kolkata: Dey's Publishers, p. 46.
Gupta R. (1999a) *Alor Abhimukhe: The Life and Times of Priyabala Gupta*, Kolkata: Dey's Publishers.
Gupta R. (1999b) *Smritimanjusha: Priyabala Gupta*, Kolkata: Dey's Publishers.
Hardgrove A. (2005) *Community and Public Culture: The Marwaris in Calcutta 1897–1997*, New York: Columbia University Press (Gutenberg E).

Harrison M. (1994) *Public Health in British India: Anglo-Indian Preventive Medicine, 1859–1914*, Cambridge: Cambridge University Press.
Hatty S. (1999) *The Disordered Body: Epidemic Disease and Cultural Transformation*, Albany: State University of New York Press.
Hofmeyr I. (2013) *Gandhi's Printing Press: Experiments in Slow Reading*, Cambridge: Harvard University Press.
India PHFI. About PHFI. Available at: https://www.phfi.org/about-us/about-phfi.
Jeffery R. (1988) *The Politics of Health in India*, Berkeley: University of California Press.
Jhabvala R.P. (1999) *Heat and Dust*, New York: Counterpoint.
Karlekar M. (1986) Kadambini and the Bhadralok: Early Debates over Women's Education in Bengal. *Economic and Political Weekly* XXI: 25–31.
Kelleher M. (1997) *The Feminization of Famine: Expressions of the Inexpressible?* Durham: Duke University Press.
Khare R.S. (1992) *The Eternal Food: Gastronomic Ideas and Influences of Hindus and Buddhists*, Albany: State University of New York Press.
Kidambi P. (2007) *The Making of the Indian Metropolis*, New York: Ashgate.
Kumar A. (1998) *Medicine and the Raj: British Medical Policy in India, 1835–1911*, New Delhi: Sage Publications.
Kumar A. (2001) *Indian Drug Industry under the Raj*, Hyderabad: Orient Longman.
Kumar D. (1997) Unequal Contenders, Uneven Ground: Medical Encounters in British India, 1820–1920. In: Cunningham A. and Andrews B. (eds) *Western Medicine as Contested Knowledge*. London: Routledge.
Lal M. (1994) The Politics of Gender and Medicine in Colonial India: The Countess of Dufferin's Fund, 1885–1888. *Bulletin for History of Medicine* 68: 29–66.
Landy J. and Saler M. (2009) *The Re-Enchantment of the World: Secular Magic in a Rational Age*, Stanford: Stanford University Press.
Lears J. (1994) *Fables of Abundance: A Cultural History of Advertising in America*, New York: Basic Books.
Liebeskind C. (2014) Arguing Science: Unani Tibb, Hakims, and Biomedicine in India, 1900–50. In: Ernst W. (ed.) *Plural Medicine, Tradition and Modernity, 1800–2000*. London and New York: Routledge.
Lupton D. (1995) *The Imperative of Health: Public Health and the Regulated Body*, Thousand Oaks, CA: Sage Publications.
Martin J. and Ramaswamy S.R. (2014) *Empires of Vision: A Reader*, Durham: Duke University Press.
McClintock A. (1995) *Imperial Leather: Race, Gender and Sexuality in the Colonial Contest*, New York: Routledge.
McLean S. (2004) *The Event and its Terrors: Ireland, Famine, and Modernity*, Stanford: Stanford University Press.
Mehta U. (1997) *Liberal Strategies of Exclusion*, Berkeley: University of California Press.
Metcalf T. (1998) *Ideologies of the Raj*, Cambridge: Cambridge University Press.

Mishra D. (1987) *Advertising in Indian Newspapers, 1780–1947*, Behrampur: Ishani Publications.
Misra A. (2004) *Public Health Issues and the Freedom Movement: Gandhi on Nutrition, Sanitation, and Infectious Diseases and Health Care*, New Delhi: Manohar Publishers and Distributors.
Morash C. (1995) *Writing the Irish Famine*, Oxford: Clarendon Press.
Mukherjee M. (1995) *Women's Work in Bengal, 1880–1930: A Historical Analysis*, Delhi: Oxford University Press.
Mukherjee M. (2011) *Churchill's Dirty War: The British Empire and the Ravaging of India During World War II*, New York: Basic Books.
Mukherjee S. (2001) *Disciplining the Body? Health Care for Women and Children in Early Twentieth Century Bengal*, New Delhi: Tulika.
Mushtaq M.U. (2009) Public Health in British India: A Brief Account of the History of Medical Services and Disease Prevention in Colonial India. *Indian Journal of Community Medicine* 34: 6–14.
Naregal V. (2001) *Language Politics, Elites, and the Public Sphere: Western India under Colonialism*, New Delhi: Permanent Black.
Office of the Superintendent. (1908) *Twenty Third Annual Report of The National Association for Supplying Female Medical Aid to the Women of India*, Calcutta: Office of the Superintendent, pp. 10–12.
Orsini F. (2002) *The Hindi Public Sphere, 1920–1940: Language and Literature in the Age of Nationalism*, Delhi: Oxford University Press.
Pahari S. (1997) *Unish Satake Banglai Sanatani Chikitsha Byabastha* (Medical Systems in Nineteenth Century Bengal), Calcutta: Progressive Publishers.
Petersen A. (1997a) *The New Public Health: Discourses, Knowledge, Strategies*, Thousand Oaks, CA: Sage Publications.
Petersen Alan and Lupton D. (1997b) *The New Public Health: Discourses, Knowledges, Strategies*, Thousand Oaks, CA: Sage Publications.
Poovey M. (1988) *Uneven Developments: The Ideological Work of Gender in Mid-Victorian England*, Chicago: University of Chicago Press.
Prasad S. (2006) Crisis, Identity, and Social Distinction: Cultural Politics of Food, Taste, and Consumption in Late Colonial Bengal. *Journal of Historical Sociology* 19: 246–265.
Preston R. (1995) *The Hot Zone: The Terrifying True Story of the Origins of the Ebola Virus*, New York: Anchor Books.
Ramagundam R. (2008) *Gandhi's Khadi: A History of Contention and Conciliation*, New Delhi: Orient Black Swan.
Ramasubban R. (1982) *Public Health and Medical Research in India: Their Origins Under the Impact of British Colonial Policy*, Stockholm: SAREC.
Ray B. (2001) *Women, Politics and Identity in Colonial Bengal, 1900–1947*, Kolkata: K.P. Bagchi and Company.
Ray K. (1998) *History of Public Health: Colonial Bengal, 1921–1947*, Calcutta: K.P. Bagchi and Company.
Ray P.C. (1936) *Anna Samasyay Bangalir Parajoy o Tahar Pratikar* (The Food Crisis, Bengali's Defeat and Its Remedy), Kolkata: Ranjan Publishing House.

Ray U. (2012) *Constructing a 'Pure' Body: The Discourse of Nutrition in Colonial Bengal*, Institute of Development Studies Occasional Paper 40.
Richards T. (1990) *The Commodity Culture of Victorian England*, Stanford: Stanford University Press.
Roy B. (1995a) *Unish Satake Deshiya Bhashai Chikitshabigyan Charcha* (The Pursuit of Medical Science in the Nineteenth Century in the Vernacular), Kolkata: Ananda Publishers.
Roy T. (1995b) *Disciplining the Printed Text: Colonial and Nationalist Surveillance of Bengali Literature*, Minneapolis: University of Minnesota Press.
Roy P. (2010) *Alimentary Tracts: Appetites, Aversions, and the Postcolonial*, Durham: Duke University Press.
Saler M. (2006) Modernity and Enchantment: A Historiographic Review. *American Historical Review* 111 (3): 692–716.
Sarkar T. (1999) *Words to Win: The Making of Amar Jiban: A Modern Autobiography*, New Delhi: Kali for Women.
Sarkar T. (2011) *Gandhi and Social Relations*, Cambridge: Cambridge University Press.
Scott P. (1998) *The Jewel in the Crown (The Raj Quartet)*, Chicago: University of Chicago Press.
Sen K.I. (1928) *Bangalir Khadya* (A Handbook on the Principles of Bengali Dietetics), Kolkata: ArogyaNiketan.
Sharma M. (2009) Creating a Consumer: Exploring Medical Advertisements in Colonial India. In: Harrison M. and Pati B. (eds) *The Social History of Health and Medicine in Colonial India*, London: Routledge.
Shetty S. (2008) *The Quack Whom We Know: Illness and Nursing in Gandhi*, London: Routledge.
Skaria A. (2010) Living by Dying. In: Anand Pandian and Daud Ali (eds) *In Ethical Life in South Asia*, Bloomington: Indiana University Press.
Smith S. and Watson J. (1998) *Women, Autobiography, Theory: A Reader*, Madison: University of Wisconsin Press.
Stage S. and Vincenti B.V. (1997) *Rethinking Home Economics: Women and the History of a Profession*, Ithaca: Cornell University Press.
Stoler A.L. (2009) *Along the Archival Grain: Epistemic Anxieties and Colonial Common Sense*, Princeton: Princeton University Press.
Suhrud T. (2011) *Gandhi's Key Writings: In Search of Unity*, Cambridge: Cambridge University Press.
Tarlo E. (1996) *Clothing Matters: Dress and Identity in India*, Chicago: University of Chicago Press.
Thrift N. (2010) Understanding the Material Practices of Glamour. In: Gregg M. and Seigworth G.J. (eds) *The Affect Theory Reader*. Durham: Duke University Press.
Tomes N. (1998) *The Gospel of Germs: Men, Women, and the Microbe in American Life*, Cambridge, MA: Harvard University Press.
Turkle S. (2007a) *Evocative Objects: Things We Think With*, Boston: MIT Press.
Turkle S. (2007b) *What Makes an Object Evocative?* Cambridge, MA: MIT Press.
Vernon J. (2007) *Hunger: A Modern History*, Cambridge, MA: Belknap Press.

Wald P. (2008) *Contagious: Cultures, Carriers, and the Outbreak Narrative*, Durham: Duke University Press.
Walsh J. (2004) *Domesticity in Colonial India*, Lanham, MD: Rowman and Littlefield.
Weisenfeld G. (2012) *Imaging Disaster: Tokyo and the Visual Culture of Japan's Great Earthquake of 1923*, Berkeley: University of California Press.
Williams R. (1993) Advertising: The Magic System. In: During S. (ed.) *The Cultural Studies Reader*, London: Routledge.

Index

Note: Locators followed by the letter 'n' refer to notes.

adulteration of food, 27–33
  embodiment in, 30
advertisement
  in colonial Bengal, 93, 96, 97, 99, 100–3, 108–11, 115
  commercial visuality, 89, 91, 93, 110, 112
  contagion of, 109–12
  enchantment, 90–3, 106, 110–11
  hygienic/beauty products, 89, 111
  Indian middle class, 90, 109–11
  late nineteenth and early twentieth century, 89–91, 95–7, 112, 114
  magazines, 97, 101–3, 105, 110
  medical, 89, 93, 96–7, 99, 100, 102
  newspaper, 90–1, 97–103, 105–7, 110
  popular journals, 90, 97, 110
  sentiments, 90, 95, 109–10
Advertising Association's Research Department, 101
Ahmed, S., 11
Akaler Sandhaney (In Search of Famine), 21, 24, 35–7
alimentary anxieties, 23–42
Alimentary Tracts: Appetites, Aversions, and the Postcolonial, 26
All India Annual Sanitary Conference, 4
All India Women's Conference (AIWC), 65
allopathic medicines, 12–13, 22, 79–80, 91, 96–7, 100, 102
Alter, J., 43–4, 47–9
Amrita Bazar Patrika, 98, 99–101
ancient land, 3–4, 8–9

Anderson, W., 117n12
anxiety, politics of, 27–33
Anyasamasya (Scarcity of Rice/Food), 31
Appadurai, A., 26, 46, 122n4
Arnold, D., 10, 13, 33, 96
Aryanari, 77
Ashani Sanket (Distant Thunder), 21, 24, 35, 37
Association of Medical Women, 64
Attewell, G., 127n22
Ayurveda, 13
Ayurvedic medicines, 12–13, 22, 80, 91, 96–7, 100–1, 103, 109

Bagchi, J., 75
Bala, P., 9, 117n14, 118n27
Bala, S., 122n17
Balfour, M.I., 124n10
Bandyopadhyay, A., 71, 124n17, 125n22
Bangalir Khadya O Pushti (1935), 31
Bangalir Khadya Samasya (Bengalis and their Food Scarcity), 31
Bangalir Khadya (The Food of Bengalis), 31
Bashford, A., 114, 129n4
Basu, A.R., 119n44, 124n14
Basu, Dr Chunilal, 73
Bayly, C. A., 31, 119n31, 119n43, 120n18
Bean, S. S., 119n31
Benckiser, Reckitt, 2
Bengal, 3–4, 9, 11–13, 15–22, 24–5, 27–42, 60–1, 63, 65–6, 73–6, 81–3, 89–91, 93, 96–7, 99–103, 105, 107–11, 113–14
  contact zones, 16

evocative objects, 15
Western medical knowledge in, 19
Bengal Chemicals and Pharmaceutical Works Limited, 13
Bengalee, 101
the Bengal Food Adulteration Act of 1919, 29
Bengali *babu*, 27
the Bengal Municipal Act of 1884, 29
Bennett, J., 93, 126n10
Berridge, V., 119n45
Betrayal of Trust: The Collapse of Global Public Health, 1
bhadralok, 27
bhadramahila, 63
Bhattacharya, N. C., 21, 24, 28, 31, 33, 38, 120n21
Bill and Melinda Gates Foundation, 2
Birla, R., 122n4, 122n5
Borthwick, M., 63, 124n4
Bose, P. K., 119n41
Brahmachari, 50
Burke, T., 94–5, 103, 126n17, 128n40
Burton, A., 55, 81, 123n21, 124n17, 125n44
Butler, Spencer Harcourt, 3, 8, 117n4
Bynum, W. F., 126n18

Campbell, D., 107, 120n9
care
   competing moralities of, 60–88
   women's writings, social-political context of, 61–6
Chakarabarty, G., 121n38
Chakrabarty, D., 118n31
Chakrabarty, H., 129n1
Chatterjee, M., 121n27
Chatterjee, P., 18, 119n39, 119n43
Chaudhurani, Saraladevi, 65
Churchill's Dirty War: The British Empire and the Ravaging of India DuringWorldWar II (2011), 28
Ciarlo, D., 89–90, 126n1

cleanliness, 5, 11–12, 17, 21–2, 45, 53, 56, 73–4, 90, 95, 102, 106, 110
clinical Christianity, 9
Cohn, B., 118n31
colonization of taste, 31
Coming Plague: Newly Emerging Diseases in a World Out of Balance, 1
contagions, 1–22, 60–88
Contagions of Empire, 16
Contagions of Feeling, 11, 16
Contagious: Cultures, Carriers, and the Outbreak Narrative, 16
Contagious Diseases Acts, 10
Cooter, R., 28, 120n10
cosmetic products, 102–3
Curried Cultures, 26

Das, S., 31, 118n26, 127n22
Dasgupta, R., 31, 39–40, 121n38
dayabal (the power of compassion), 50
Deb, C., 81, 123n2, 125n46, 126n54
Debi, P., 61, 67, 69–71, 78, 81–8, 125n21, 125n47
degree of urgency, 4
Demon in the Freezer, 1
Desivilliar, R. C., 124n11
Dettol *Surakshit Parivar*, 2
Devi, Swarnakumari, 65
Devji, F., 122n4
Diet and Diet Reform, 21
Dube, S., 92, 126n6
Dufferin Fund, 62
Dyson, L., 72, 125n26

Eaton, N., 121n37
embodiment, 6, 23–33, 49, 80
Emerging Infectious Diseases, 2
Empires of Hygiene, 16
Epstein, H., 129n3
Ernst, W., 127n18
Eternal Food: Gastronomic Ideas and Experiences of Hindus and Buddhists, 26

famine, 18, 21, 24–5, 27–9, 33–42
Farquhar, J., 120n2
fasting, 43, 48, 50–1
Festa, L., 109, 129n49
Fisher, J, 30, 120n17
Fitzgerald, R., 117n13
food and body, histories of, 26–7
food and hunger, affect in, 23–42
Forbes, G., 63, 123n1, 124n3, 124n7, 124n17
Forbes, Geraldine, 63
Foucault, M., 119n34

Gandhi, M., 15, 21, 43–59
  body and affect, 46–50
  contagion, medicine as, 56–9
  fasting and, 50–2
  race and politics of hygiene, 52–6
Gandhi's Body: Sex, Diet, and the Politics of Nationalism, 47
Ganguly, K., 63, 65, 71
Gigliotti, S., 125n23
Global Hygiene Council, 2
Goldman, R., 109, 129n48
Gonsalves, P., 118n31
Good Life, 50
Greenough, P., 34, 121n31
Gregg, M., 118n23
Grihasthamangal, 103–4
Guha, S., 120n20
Gupta, P., 62, 69–71, 75–81, 84–5, 88, 125n33
Gupta, R., 70, 124n17, 125n20

hakimi treatment, 12, 22, 97, 101
Hanson, M., 120n2
Hardgrove, A., 30, 120n15
Harrison, M., 117n8, 118n16
Hatty, S., 28, 120n8
Hind Swaraj, 1909, 45–6, 56–7
Hofmeyr, I., 54, 122n19, 123n25
homeopathy, 13, 96, 101
Hooker, C., 114, 129n4
Hot Zone: A Terrifying True Story, 1
Hunger: A Modern History, 41
Hungry Bengal, 21

hygiene
  affective history, 5–17
  awareness, 2
  colonialism and, 5–11
  contagion and, 6
  cultural politics of, 1–22
  emergence of, 5
  feeling and, 6
  genealogy of, 3
  Mahatma Gandhi and, 43–59
  methods and sources, 17–20
  objects of, 11–17
hygiene and beauty products
  advertisement, 89, 93, 102, 111
  clientele, 89–90
  commodification, 90, 95, 105
  domains and concerns, 102–5
  gendered nature, 90, 95–6, 102–3, 105–6, 108–11

IMS, *see* Indian Medical Service (IMS)
Indian Medical Service (IMS), 7
Indian Opinion, 21, 45

Jeffery, R., 118n27
Jhabvala, R. P., 120n11
jitakshara, 69
Joshee, Anandibai, 62

Kabya Kusumanjali, 77
Kanakanjali, 77
Karlekar, M., 123n2, 124n17
Kelleher, M., 35, 121n33
Key to Health, 21, 43–5, 49
Khadya (Food), 31
Khadya Tattwa (Treatise on Food), 31
Khare, R.S., 120n3
Kidambi, P., 10, 118n21
Kosambi, M., 62
Kumar, A., 10, 97, 118n18, 118n28, 127n19, 127n25
Kumar, D., 127n22

Lady Chelmsford All India League for Maternity and Child Welfare, 64

Lal, M., 62, 123n1
Lancet, 1
Landy, J., 91, 126n2
Lears, J., 108, 128n42, 129n46
A Lesson From The Plague, 55
Liebeskind, C., 127n22
Lifebuoy Men, 95, 104
Living by Dying, 50
Lock hospitals, 10
Loughlin, K., 119n45
Lupton, D., 15, 119n35, 119n45
Lux Women, 95, 104

Martin, J., 94
McClintock, A., 94–5, 126n16, 129n46
McLean, S., 33, 121n28, 121n35
medical consumerism, 12, 90
medical ideologies, 101–2, 114
medical marketplace, 12–14, 22, 90, 93, 96–7, 100, 101, 108, 110
medical profession, 62–3, 80, 105
Mehta, U., 8, 117n11
Meike, W., 122n17
Metcalf, T., 8, 117n11
midwives, 63–4, 79, 105
Mishra, D., 127n24
Misra, A., 122n7, 123n28
Modi, N., 52
Mone Pare, 81–3, 85–6
Morash, C., 34, 121n30, 121n35
Mukherjee, M., 28, 120n7, 124n6
Mukherjee, S., 124n12
Municipal Amendment Act of 1917, 29
Mushtaq, M. U., 118n22

Naregal, V., 119n38
National Advertising Agency, 101
New England Journal of Medicine, 1
Nightingale, Florence, 10
N.N. Sen and Company Private Limited, 13
non-Bengali communities, 27, 31

Orsini, F., 119n38

Pahari, S., 118n25, 127n20
paradoxes, 5, 23–4, 54, 80, 91
patent medicines, 18, 89, 97, 99
Pather Alo ('Leading Lights'), 61, 66–70, 72, 74
pathogenic, 10, 113–14
personal sanitation, awareness of, 2
Petersen, A., 119n45, 125n30
PHFI, *see* the Public Health Foundation of India (PHFI)
plague (1896–1897), 10
Poovey, M., 10, 118n18, 118n19
Porter, R., 126n18
post-HIV, 7
Prasad, S., 120n16, 120n19
Preston, R., 1, 117n1
Priyabala Gupta, 78
Public Culture, 46
public health, narratives of, 6
Public Health Foundation of India (PHFI), 2

Ramagundam, R., 118n31
Ramasubban, R., 9, 118n15
Ramaswamy, S. R., 94, 126n13
'ramzan' fast, 51
    see also fasting
Ray, B., 124n13, 124n14
Ray, K., 118n20, 120n12
Ray, P.C., 120n22
Ray, U., 32, 121n22
Raychaudhuri, T., 124n3, 124n17
Richards, T., 94–5, 126n14
Roy, B., 20, 127n21
Roy, P., 26, 120n5
Roy, T., 119n40

Sakhi Samiti, 65
Saler, M., 91–2, 126n2, 126n4
sanitary awakening, 3–4, 8
Sarkar, S., 13, 96, 118n26, 127n21
Sarkar, T., 49, 69, 78, 122n11, 124n16
satyagraha, 21, 43, 50, 52
satyagrahi, 50
Scott, P., 120n11

Seigworth, G. J., 118n23, 118n24
Sen, A., 124n17
Sen, K. I., 127n26
Sentimental Figures of Empire in Eighteenth-Century Britain and France (Festa), 109
Sharma, M., 100, 127n27, 127n30
Shetty, S., 123n29
Sishu-O-Matri Mangal Kendra (Centre for theWelfare of Children and Mothers), 66
Skaria, A., 50, 122n13
Smith, S., 125n18, 125n43
Smritimanjusha (A Treasury of Memories), 62, 75, 77–8, 80–1
somatic nationalism, 14
Stage, S., 129n53
The *Statesman*, 101
Stoler, A.L., 6, 117n5
The Story of My Experiments with Truth, 1925 (Mahatma Gandhi), 21, 43–5, 48, 58
Suhrud, T., 122n3
Swachh Bharat Campaign, 52
swadeshi, 21, 31, 76
Swaraj, 43–59

Tarde, Gabriel, 15
Tarlo, E., 118n31
Tea and Food Adulteration, 1834–75, 30
technology of self, 43
therapeutic chaos, 14
Thrift, N., 15, 119n32
Times of India, 54
Tomes, N., 129n53
Turkle, S., 15, 119n32, 125n29

Unani, 13, 20

Vernon, J., 41, 119n38, 121n42
Victoria Memorial Scholarship Fund, 64
Vincenti, B. V., 129n53

Wald, P., 7, 10, 16, 117n9, 118n23
Walsh, J., 119n37
Weisenfeld, G., 121n34
Williams, R., 129n45
Women's Indian Association (WIA), 65

Young, R., 124n10

zenana, 62

GPSR Compliance

The European Union's (EU) General Product Safety Regulation (GPSR) is a set of rules that requires consumer products to be safe and our obligations to ensure this.

If you have any concerns about our products, you can contact us on

ProductSafety@springernature.com

In case Publisher is established outside the EU, the EU authorized representative is:

Springer Nature Customer Service Center GmbH
Europaplatz 3
69115 Heidelberg, Germany

www.ingramcontent.com/pod-product-compliance
Lightning Source LLC
Chambersburg PA
CBHW071614100426
42873CB00004B/42